Dorth...

Thank you
for being an
amazing mother
and support.

The
Chem-HO

I am so
proud to meet
you.

ally

ALLY LANE

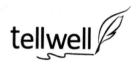

Tellwell Talent
www.tellwell.ca

ISBN
978-1-77370-371-8 (Hardcover)
978-1-77370-370-1 (Paperback)
978-1-77370-372-5 (eBook)

CHAPTER 1
The Ass-Man

You know that expression: "Let's take it from the top"? In my case, let's take it from the bottom – rock bottom. Allow me to set the scene. I'm thirty-eight years old and single. I should stress, STILL single; never married. No kids. My last relationship was four years ago with a very modest man who had big dreams of becoming an ass model. No, not a butt model showing off his gluteus maximums in a nice pair of Levis, but a naked, bare ass, model. He made a calendar using pictures of his naked ass standing in front of different monuments, one for each month of the year. He sold his calendar at flea markets and at my family reunion. I was devastated when he dumped me to take his sweet cheeks overseas. I thought he was The One. I wanted him to be The One. I NEEDED him to be The One. I couldn't take another day of being referred to as "The old single one". I thought we were the perfect couple: I hated my butt, and he loved his.

Here I am four years later in the same bar where I had met The Ass-man. Oh, I'm not insulting him. That is what he called himself. Only this time, I am a little worse for wear. I'm sitting alone at the bar, sharing the last stool with a couple that is making out. I've already been warned by the bartender that I'll be cut off if I keep singing the Three's Company theme song, but I can't help it. I'm drinking a bottle of Merlot through a straw, straight from the bottle. Let me explain.

Due to a recent accident, my hands are in full casts, right up to my elbows. I can't grip a glass to save my life. "Completely shattered," the doctor had explained. I don't know if she was talking about my mental state or my bones but at this point, they're interchangeable. I broke them both a week ago, on a date with a boy 15 years my junior named Rob. You could say that our version of foreplay was standing on the edge of a cliff face, on mountain bikes, overlooking a seesaw, which I thought I could land on while remaining intact on the bike seat. Instead, I landed in an ambulance sucking on laughing gas to numb the pain, which by the way, I highly recommend.

This incident was the grand finale of a three month long detox from dating that I had crowned the "No Bang Theory". I had finally thrown in the towel and decided to give up on finding The One. In fact, I had completely given up on finding anyone. I could no longer compartmentalize between love, sex, and George Clooney. I had been labeled crazy by more than a dozen lovers and I had started to believe that Gnarls Barkely was singing about me: "I remember when, I remember, I remember when I lost my mind."

See, when my breakup with The Ass-man landed me in extensive counselling, both in a professional therapist's office and in a wine bar down the block, I started begging for answers. My therapist explained to me that: "When a woman has sex, she releases a chemical that is harder to kick than an addiction to heroin." Oh great! And I thought I had escaped the grunge era with nothing more than a plaid shirt and knowing every line to the movie Singles. Alas, (yes, I used alas), my therapist was right. I decided to look into this further and I discovered that this chemical is the same one that a mother releases when she gives birth, which makes her physically bound to her baby. So I realized that when I was having sex, I felt emotionally bound to my various lovers or, in some instances, just bound. Handcuffs were on sale at the costume shop.

No wonder I keep falling in love with every man I date. In my twenties I dated a sex addict for over a year. I was convinced I could change him. He was convinced that having a threesome with his boss and his wife was the best way to get a promotion. I also had an on and off relationship with a guy who, while breaking up with me stated, "I only date girls that look like Meg Ryan and you don't look like her". It has taken me years to get over that one. It has also taken me years to learn every line from: When Harry met Sally. My dating history spans from men who can't pay a phone bill to men who phone the wrong girlfriend. The common thread they all have was my love and dedication to them all. It wasn't my fault. It was "the chemicals".

At the time, all of my friends and family were matched up or married with kids. It was at that point that I decided I couldn't continue releasing "the chemicals" all over town. I felt like the main character in a single woman's apocalypse. It was time to make a change: no sex whatsoever, including masturbation. It was crunch time. I had to stop the pattern. Getting no business was serious business. But my "No Bang Theory" came to a literal screaming halt when I fell off the wagon. I thought the best way to forget about sex was to hop on a plane and head for the biggest party in the world, Dublin on St. Patrick's Day. Nobody is horny surrounded by tourists, drinking for twelve hours straight, right? Wrong. It is like Vegas with leprechauns. My transgression happened with a 21 year old tourist from Italy named Fabio on the lobby sofa at a discount hotel. Receiving attention from a much younger man felt good, really good. Or maybe it was the memory foam? From the moment I fell off of that lobby sofa to the floor, I realized that the secret was not in refraining. The secret was the receiving the attention from much younger men. It suddenly hit me that dating much younger men meant that there was no pressure because I didn't have to envision a future with them. It meant I could stop putting deadlines on my future and just enjoy life. It was that moment on the lobby floor that I decided that getting married and having children was not in the cards for me. I would rather enjoy the wild ride of dating than set unrealistic expectations for myself. I was having a blast: until I broke both hands.

His name was Rob and he was an Australian bartender in Canada on a work Visa. I was on a girl's weekend at a mountain resort challenging all of my stay-at-home mom friends to another body shot. I don't know if it was my expertise in funnelling tequila through a set of double D's or the fact that I tipped him twenty-five percent, but Rob took a liking to me. After exchanging numbers I went back home and he went back to juggling bottles of flavoured vodka. A few days later he texted me: "What are you doing?" Without even thinking, I responded: "What are you wearing?" I don't know exactly what answer I was expecting but my quick response had instigated a weeklong sexting conversation that would make a porn star blush. I knew there was no future with Crocodile Dundee Jr. so I thought I would have a little fun. Finally his blue balls got the best of him and he said: "I need to see you." Looking back, I should have texted him a photo of me in a push up bra and then blocked his number. Instead, I got in my car and drove three hours to get my 'shrimp on the bar-bee'. I don't even know what that means, so this is your chance to insert your own Aussie sex pun.

I met him at the ski hill on a hot July day. He thought it would be fun to go downhill mountain biking. This is an extreme sport where you ride the chairlift up and ride your bike down over obstacles and jumps graded from 'easy' to 'I don't have a mortgage to pay so I don't care if I live or die'. On our final descent, he chose the latter. The run was called Crazytrain. I should have sensed the irony. There was a massive sign blocking the entrance that warned, "Extreme Caution. If staring down this run scares you, DO NOT ATTEMPT." Yep, it scared me. It was the scariest moment of my life, equivalent to seeing my brother naked. Gross.

I told my date I didn't want to do it. He insisted I could. This banter went back and forth for five minutes. I argued my case and he rolled his eyes until finally he said: "If you do this stunt, I'll have sex with you." That was it. Before I could say, desperate, my bike was barrelling off of a six-foot cliff and my body was slamming onto the wooden plank below. There was no question that I was badly hurt. I just didn't know how badly. My hands got caught in the tiny opening of the wooden seesaw, and the weight of my body had carried me over myself and pried my hands until the bones literally snapped. I was in such shock that I started to vomit and the first thing that came to my mind was "Are we still going to have sex?" My young Aussie fantasy had come to a staggering halt as I lay screeching in the back of the ambulance. I spent the next three days in hospital and Rob spent it on magic mushrooms with an age appropriate Swedish tourist.

Do you know that you can't do anything without properly functioning hands? Think about it for a second;

driving, texting, brushing your hair, brushing your teeth, peeling an orange and peeling your clothes off in an amateur strip contest. I thought to myself, "What was the meaning behind this accident? Why did it happen to me?" My friend Sarah told me: "It means to stop whatever you are doing because it's not working." Hmmm. Ya think so? This ended my brief stint as a cougar. I immediately went back to being single.

So here I am at the bar with my straw and bottle, my friend Sarah is at the far end chatting up a set of twins. She's so talented at chatting people up. I wish I had that gift. I wish I wasn't stuck here with their "gay male friend" telling him all about my dildo. It's too bad he's gay. He's quite handsome with deep-set brown eyes and an olive complexion. He looks like Danny from The Mindy Project except shorter. I wish I could give him some sort of hand signal to go away but I can't, I have two broken hands. Right now all I can think about is: how did I get here? I don't mean how I physically got to this bar at this moment. I'm not that drunk, yet. Maybe I am? Wait, did I just pee myself? No, it's more of a: "How did my life become this? Haven't I been through enough? Haven't I paid my dues?" I mean, three years ago, I even went through breast cancer. Can the universe throw me a bone here or at least a refill?

CHAPTER 2
Butt Lift and Broncos

It was October of 2008 and I was lying in bed, alone in the dark, alone, contemplating about how I could finally stop this endless cycle of: lying in bed, alone, contemplating about being in bed, alone. I had recently started a job teaching at a prestigious acting school inspiring hopefuls in dealing with the 'dog eats dog' world of the industry when really, the only world I knew how to deal with was the 'teacher eats an entire family size KFC bucket in the bathroom.' The truth was, I could teach them about acting but I wasn't equipped to share my knowledge about dealing with rejection. I was in my mid-thirties and I couldn't even persuade my own dog to sleep at the foot of my bed.

The Ass-Man had moved out fifteen months prior and in a state of vengeful spite, I demanded he take the bed with him. What a dumb move! I had to resort to sleeping in a single bed in the spare room. My life is full of ironies; that, and empty bottles of Merlot.

The phone rang, and for a brief moment, I thought: maybe it is Ass-Man calling to apologize? Now, most women fantasize about a topless Channing Tatum galloping up on a white horse with a family size bucket of KFC, but my weekly fantasy was an ex, returning, grovelling for forgiveness. Let's make it clear, I didn't want him back, I just wanted him to acknowledge the way he had treated me. Or maybe, I just wanted him to acknowledge ME? Could it be? Sometimes a complex internal issue can be traced back to one simple thing. Could this be it? Or did I want him to make a viral video crying out my name? Maybe.

Prior to meeting him, I had a lot of issues with my throat. I was consistently losing my voice and lived off of lozenges and an unhealthy relationship with WebMD. It was terrifying because I relied on my voice for work and if I lost it, I couldn't work. Being a self-employed actor with a mortgage and no health benefits may not have been the wisest career choice, but for me, it was the only choice. Acting made me feel whole, alive and happy. I made my living playing make believe. It was a no brainer.

I used to spend a lot of my time networking in an entrepreneur's club with people who were so busy trying to get ahead that they never let me speak or express my ideas. When I voiced my concern about my throat to my doctor she said: "Do you feel like nobody listens to you?" My heart sank and tears welled up immediately. She was right. I spent the majority of my time trying to get attention from these unimportant people and I was pushing my voice through my throat. I didn't need medical help. I needed to stop surrounding myself with multi-level marketing groups that promised me a fulfilling life if I bought their $800 face cream. I wonder if all I want from my ex is to be acknowledged. Was she right? Nah!!! He's a douche.

The phone was still ringing. Geez, who was calling? Hadn't they heard of Facebook Messenger, or a Sunday morning hangover? I remember not being able to see the damn phone. I thought I'd better turn on a light. As I stretched out my arms to reach for the light, my thumb grazed over a new mole on my chest. This one felt larger than usual. I know because I feel my boobs up a lot, and down, and all around. It's another thing to remove; like that stack of Brazilian Butt Lift DVD's sitting on the bookshelf. I wasted 'three easy payments' on only a slight shifting.

Before I could make out the entire number, I could see it is a call from Winnipeg. Yes, you read that right, Winnipeg. No, it's not the fictional place you hear about on American sitcoms; the place they call out to get a laugh. It is an actual city in the middle of Canada. Winnipeg is where I grew up, went to university, and learned all of life's valuable lessons including how to make myself faint in the hall as my mother, clueless, walked by singing Tony Orlando.

My mother is a very sweet petite woman with the voice of a tea kettle that has been on high boil. I would leave the house for school and I could hear what sounded like Edith Bunker singing: "Tie a Yellow Ribbon Round the Old Oak Tree" from six blocks away. She grew up very poor and doesn't hesitate to remind me of this every chance she gets. She is the only person I have ever met that has bought a coupon book, with a coupon. Once she bought me a cup of coffee. A day later I received an invoice, with interest.

My dad is a hardworking man with a dry sense of humour. He resembles Newman from Seinfeld but has the heart of John Candy. He is uber smart with a photographic memory and the mathematical brain of a robot. His job titles have ranged from CEO, to CFO to C3PO. His brain, however, is missing the part that tells him how to dress. He wears the same pair of pyjama pants day in and day out. One of my fondest memories is of him wearing them so much that the elastic had stretched out to triple his waist size. He didn't ever bother to fix them. He just held the pants up in a ball and walked around the house like that, for fifteen years.

My parents raised four children. You know the old saying that everything comes in threes? Well, in our case, it was twos; two girls, two boys, all two years apart. My eldest sister Lisa is the smart one. I am the dramatic one. My brother Matt is the king of the nerds, even before it became hip. Yep, I used the description 'hip'. I just sounded like a grandparent. You know what I mean about nerds though, right? Today it's cool to like fantasy novels and Live Action Role Playing. In the late eighties, Matt would stage scenes from Monty Python at the back of the city bus. He kept the passengers entertained. You know people like your stuff when they simultaneously roll their eyes and then get off the bus nine stops early, right? He was so ahead of his time.

Rounding out the Lane clan is my brother Andy. Andy is the youngest child, adopted out of the Special Needs Program in 1976, although it took almost twenty-four years to get a proper diagnosis as to what his special need was. He attended regular school but never completed an entire year due to behavioural problems. He reached fame long before I did; gracing the front cover of the local paper wearing a handmade glove out of my mother's kitchen knives and duct tape. He looked like the psychotic version of Edward Scissorhands. The caption read: <u>Suburban Gangs Invade the Streets of Winnipeg</u>. Not only did we have an eleven-year old gang leader living in our house, my mom had no cutlery. Andy used the rest of the knives to carve inspirational messages into the dining room table. My morning pick me up ranged from "Burn in Hell" to "I Love Sluts".

We all dealt with my brother's behaviour in different ways. It wasn't easy living with the neighbourhood psychopath. My sister would bury her head in books, Dad in his work, Matt in his Dungeons and Dragons, my mom in her tears. Me? I used my imagination. All of my fantasies involved George Clooney, an Oscar and a restraining order.

The phone was still ringing. I picked it up and it was Matt's wife, Jen. At the time, my siblings were all married with children. I was STILL the only single one. My life partner was my dog, Peggy. She was a twelve-year old Labrador nearing the end of her life. She coughed so much

I would often mistake her for Marge Simpson. I don't know where the cough came from. I sometimes imagined waking up in the middle of the night to find her smoking a pipe working out to my Butt Lift videos.

"Have you donated to my run yet?" Jen asked. She was participating in the Breast Cancer Run. She was running for a friend's sister who had been diagnosed at age twenty-seven.

"No, not yet. When is it?"

"It's today Allison. You've got ten minutes left to donate online."

The thing was that I had no direct affiliation with breast cancer. I didn't know anyone that had it. I had never even done a breast check, unless you consider duct taping my boobs to enhance my cleavage. Those women running around in pink annoyed me. But my sister-in-law needed my support, so I would support her. Plus, I needed to get out of bed. I had to pee. I swore that if I got another UTI I was going to stop wearing the same underwear for a week.

"Ok I guess I'll get up then." I hung up the phone and pulled the sheets off. My thumb grazed over the mole again. Only this time it didn't feel like a mole. I was lying on my back and looked down. I touched the spot again to feel a lump right under my right breast sticking to my rib cage. A wave of heat went through my entire body. I thought it had to be in my imagination. We were just talking about breast cancer and there was no way I could have just felt a lump. I touched it again. It was definitely there. It was hard and felt about the size of a marble, and it moved. I could move it from side to side, up and down. I started to panic. I began to check both my breasts but I had no idea what I was doing. My friend, Sue, used to email me a breast check reminder every month and I would just delete it. She was a schoolteacher and would email reminders about everything: turn off your water, set your clocks back and change your underwear. Now I wish I would have read them.

I knew I had to rub my breasts in a circle. I lay there rubbing and rubbing, but nothing was happening except static electricity and a new masturbation idea. I needed to know how to do it right and I was accomplishing nothing lying in bed rubbing my boobs together. I ran upstairs and googled it. Big mistake! In one click I had either yellow fever or an addiction to sedatives. Then I remembered that a few years earlier my mother had found a lump. I picked up the phone and called her. As soon as I heard her voice, I started to cry. I don't know if I was crying about the lump or the fact that she sounded so much like Edith Bunker.

"What's wrong dear? Have you been dumped again?"

"No, I'm not even dating anyone."

"How about joining a bridge league?"

"Mother, I found a lump."

"What do you mean? Like a lump of coal? I don't understand."

"No, on my breast, err... under my breast... I'm scared mom."

"Oh there's no reason to be scared, it's nothing."

That's the good thing about mom. Beneath her Edith exterior, she is hard as nails. She has an approach to life resembling that of an army sergeant. She is the masculine one in the relationship. I don't know how many times I have seen her tell my father to stop crying and eat his vegetables.

"Do you remember when I found a lump?" she asked sweetly.

"Yes," I replied.

"And all I had was fibrocystic breasts. Your sister has them too. That's all it is." I took a deep breath and my entire body relaxed. Oh thank God.

After that my mother changed the subject. She reminded me now that she went over budget on my birthday present. She would need a cheque from me for the difference. "You owe me five dollars."

I called my doctor the next day and told her I had found a lump and I thought it was just a cyst. "Can you be here in half an hour?" she asked. 30 minutes later, I arrived at her office and checked in with the receptionist.

"She's expecting you," she said robotically, fixated on Facebook.

Suddenly everything felt like it was happening so fast. I have waited in line for the bathroom at a Justin Beiber concert longer. And don't laugh at The Beibs, his concerts are amazing! The doctor asked me to take off my top and examined my breasts.

"My mom and my sister both have fibrocystic breasts."

"Ok," she said.

"So I must have it too."

"Maybe," she answered.

Maybe? That wasn't convincing. Maybe is something you say when you don't want to do anal. Maybe? What kind of answer was that?

"That's probably all it is, but we need to do a mammogram just to be sure."

"Ugh" I responded.

Three days later, I was getting my first mammogram. I had to stand there frozen, not allowed to move an inch while my boobs were pancaked between two giant plates. I looked down and my tits were being flattened like a grilled cheese on a George Foreman Grill. From biopsy to ultrasound, I breezed through all of these procedures knowing full well it was routine protocol. After the first week, I had shown my tits to more people than a lonely girl at Mardi Gras. That was fun, by the way.

The truth was I thought I couldn't get cancer. First of all, there is no family history of the disease. Secondly, I was always careful to take good care of myself. I HAD to. I lived alone, had a mortgage, and was self-employed. I knew that if I got sick, there was nobody to take care of me. How would I pay my bills? There was certainly no way I could move back to Winnipeg and I also felt like my life had not begun. I just paid for a year subscription to E-Harmony.

I couldn't put my parents through another Lane family crisis. Growing up, we were like those families with problems you would see on Oprah. The only difference is our problems could fit into ANY show she had on the air.

In those days, the neighbours got a new live show every week. Now, when the average cigarette smoker craves a cigarette, they may bite their nails or chew gum or even go through the ashtray for butts. When my brother Andy craves a cigarette, he goes big! It doesn't matter when or where you are. When Andy craves a smoke, it becomes a family responsibility.

He usually doesn't wake up until six in the evening. So at 4 in the morning when everyone is sleeping, Andy is on his 15th smoke of the day. When he runs out, has no money, and the corner store is closed, he calls my parents.

"Dad... Dad I need twenty bucks."

"It's four o'clock in the morning," my dad would answer.

"Give me twenty bucks."

"Goodnight Andy."

"If you don't give me money right now, I'm gonna take it all away. I'm gonna take your house away," he screamed.

That was not very threatening coming from Andy, considering he was on welfare with a grade eight education. What could he do really? There would be lawyer's fees, court battles; it would drag on longer than the American election.

So Dad hung up. But Andy was on the edge you see, and when my brother says: "I'm going to take your house away" he means take your house away, literally. That boy needed a smoke badly. Half an hour later the entire neighbourhood was awoken by the sound of tires screeching and an engine revving. There was Andy, in this Ford Bronco, with a giant chain attached on one end to the trailer hitch, and at the other to the front porch. He was literally going to try to pull the house away. The neighbours came out with their lawn chairs and morning coffees.

"What's going on this time?"

"The Lane kid is back. He's trying to pull their house away."

"What kind of chain is that? I don't think that's going to work."

"He is making a huge mess. Didn't they just have their lawn done? I should give them my landscaper's number."

"What kind of coffee is this? It's good."

"Ah, there goes their fence. That's going to cost them."

My mother was screaming, the dog was barking, the neighbours were watching, and there was Andy trying to pull the house away with his monster truck tires and bumper sticker that reads: evil is an art form.

Andy is yelling out the Bronco window, "I want my twenty dollars."

The Bronco was the same vehicle that O.J. Simpson drove years earlier in the epic car chase broadcast around the world. They stopped making the Bronco after that and renamed the vehicle "The Escape". He backed up and tried to pull it again.

"Give me twenty bucks," he demanded as the neighbours watched in horror. My parents just stood there. My mother started crying.

"Oh look Gail is out here. I'm supposed to play bridge with her tomorrow."

Now as parents, it's good to stand your ground, good to be firm, not give in. In this case, my parents should have just given in. The boy needed a smoke. My dad walked out of the house, unhooked the chain and opened his wallet. Then, my brother drove off. The neighbours folded up their chairs.

"Well that was interesting."

"Yep, I guess I'll see you next week."

"And can you bring this coffee again? It's terrific."

My parents slowly began to cut Andy off and then I became his crutch. I was finally beginning to fully understand what he had put them through all of those years. In the summer of 2006, I received an email from Andy while my parents were out of town.

It read: "July 1st is the breaking point."

Andy always has a habit of doing this. Short, vague emails with one-line statements: the end is near; I fought the law; I love sluts. But the emails about July 1st were particularly disturbing.

"July 1st is the day it all changes. Watch out on July 1st."

I became really spooked. What was going to happen on July 1st? I called my parents. They were away on some couples therapy retreat with Dr. S. until June 30th. Oh God! I called my other siblings and they didn't answer. I tried for days but couldn't get a hold of anyone. I was in a panic. I couldn't sleep. What the hell was Andy planning? He was going to kill my parents. I was convinced. Oh my God!

I started stocking up on pepper spray, added extra locks to my door, and I seriously considered buying some items from Andy's ninja catalogue. When he was a child, he had his own business selling homemade ninja weapons door to door. The business went under when one of our neighbours called the police when she found him on her roof doing cartwheels in a black cape.

On July 1st I was in Banff on business. As I sat in the bar with my cell phone next to me, I waited for it to ring. I was waiting for the "Big News". I kept looking at the television to see if The Lane Family Circus made it to prime time. Nothing came up. Later on that night, I rushed to check my email and there it was.

"Ally, I couldn't hide my anger any longer. I had to do it. I faced the facts. I told Mom and Dad. I am gay. I know they are angry and will want to rid me of their lives, but it had to be done."

That's it??? That's the breaking point?? He's gay? A few days later, I got a hold of my dad and asked him about that fateful day.

"Dad what did you think of July 1st. Are you okay?"

"What do you mean?"

"I mean the breaking point? I mean the Big Day?"

There was a pause.

"What big day?"

"Andy called you and said he was gay."

"Oh yah, I forgot about that."

"Andy sounded so upset. What exactly did you say to him?"

"I told him that was fine, as long as he kept his room clean."

Dad said that after all Andy has put us through, he being gay is nothing. Who cares? Could you imagine if all parents reacted that way when their children came out of the closet? Everybody would be gay!

I guess Andy became so mad when he didn't get the reaction or the attention he wanted with his big announcement that he came out of the closet and re-entered within four hours. He started dating a woman two days later.

So you see my parents had been through enough. It was bad enough I was single. I couldn't be single with cancer. There was no way I was going to let that happen. And then, it did.

On October 26, 2008 I got my answer. I was diagnosed with breast cancer. The treatment plan was extensive; surgeries, chemotherapy, radiation and medication. I had just received the shock of my life. I have cancer.

CHAPTER 3
Another World

Dealing with trauma, for me, is like dealing with constipation. It happens, but you know it won't last forever. I know what you may be thinking: "How dare you minimize trauma?" Or you may even be thinking, "I should have bought the Amy Schumer book instead." The truth is that I went through a lot of ordeals growing up. It arrived fiscally like a cold sore. I knew that as soon as I would get over one crisis, another one was coming and I couldn't do anything to stop it. I, therefore, had to learn some tools to deal with trauma from a very young age.

You've already received the low-down on my youngest brother. Even though he is a headache to deal with, like one of those migraines you get after day-drinking in your forties, I do love him a great deal. But another ingredient in my childhood trauma cocktail was a man dripping vodka; he was my paternal grandfather, an alcoholic. He was sentenced to prison for sexually abusing me and countless others. Whoa! Where did that come from? Now you must be REALLY regretting not buying the Amy Schumer book. I will not traumatize you with the details. After all these years, it remains a taboo subject. No child should have to endure that. Most kids spend their spare time going to birthday parties or finding ways to save for a new toy. My spare time consisted of meetings with social workers, attending court cases and giving statements to the police. I do want to express how heartbreaking this was to my parents, especially my Father. He felt he didn't protect me when I was young, so he spent his entire life trying to make up for it. I never blamed him or anyone for what happened. I realized I was just a child and could not articulate my circumstance. My dad is now in his 70s and finally letting go of the past. He is at last happy and enjoying his life. I am so proud of him. I had to learn from a very early age the value of resilience. It has shaped me into the person I am. So when cancer struck, I knew I could handle it. I had been through so much worse at such a young age. Though as a child, I was too young to articulate my disgust with my abuser, so I chose not to speak at all.

You know the kid hiding in the corner at school? That was me. Most teachers send the kid to the corner for punishment but for me, it was my sanctuary. I cried at school every day. I wasn't being bullied. I just liked to cry; it feels good. This has not changed. A stiff breeze goes by and I'm hyperventilating with tears.

Mom would receive a daily report from my teacher: "Today was a good day. She only cried once." School outings were a no go. While the entire student body was on a field trip to a cheese factory, I got to stay at home with my mom and watch Another World. I remember those days fondly. I was fascinated with soap operas. It made my life seem so normal. I even persuaded my mom to cut my hair like Linda Dano's. That didn't work out so well, though I looked more like the head of a Q-Tip.

My parents were extremely worried about my future. It did not look bright. How could I function as an adult hiding in a corner crying? They were convinced that I was destined to work in a cubicle selling magazine subscriptions. I realized that that job doesn't exist anymore, so now I've been downsized; even more reason to cry.

In the third grade, things did not improve. The teachers had arranged a special activity day where the students chose a program they had never experienced before. Out of all the choices, my mom encouraged me to try Drama. No, that's wrong. She didn't encourage me; she forced me. She looked like Joan Crawford standing above me with the permission slip. "You're doing Drama God…dam… damn it. No more wire hangers". Okay, I guess you didn't see Mommy Dearest, but it's a good reference.

On the day of Drama class, I was surprisingly calm. My mom had compared the class to what the actors do on the soap operas. So I closed my eyes and imagined I had amnesia, was possessed by the devil, and was the illegitimate daughter of an oil tycoon. The teacher made us all stand in a line and close our eyes. She instructed us to become different animals trapped in different situations. She wanted us to use our bodies and our imaginations to really immerse ourselves into that world. I absolutely loved it. I wasn't that shy little girl anymore. I was a bear stuck in honey, a bird trapped in a cage, a dog eating its own vomit. I felt free. I felt unleashed. I was taken away from my hurricane of a childhood and I didn't have to be ME anymore. I could be whatever I wanted to be. I had finally been given permission to express myself in a place of non-judgment. I was instantly hooked. Before the day came to an end, my teacher called my mother and said: "Get that girl into Drama classes".

From that moment on, I went from the girl that couldn't talk, to the girl that wouldn't shut up. I had found my passion. I started writing plays in the fourth grade. By the seventh grade, I was directing the entire student body in year-end productions. I went to extracurricular acting classes, acting camps; anything I could get my overly dramatic hands on.

I also realized it was easier to laugh than it was to cry. When a painful moment hit, I looked for the humour in it. Some moments were harder than others, like getting my period for the first time. It took me six months to discover that the cardboard around the tampon needed to be removed. Bad visual? Imagine how I felt. Pain can be funny. Really funny, and I had a lot of funny moments to get through.

So on October 26, 2008, when I walked into the doctor's office, I was prepared to laugh. First of all, the doctor knew me as Patient #48265. Getting my name remotely correct was not on her priorities list. Secondly, my dad had flown out to be with me and was wearing a new pair of 'I Love Golf' pyjama pants. This was ironic since he hadn't played golf since 1976.

"Hello Alicia. My name is Doctor Anderson. Andrea, you have a very aggressive form of breast cancer. Since you chose not to have your breasts removed, we will have to take every precaution possible so that it doesn't come back. Chemotherapy and radiation followed by another year of chemo, then five years of medication and after that, you'll have to check in every six months for the rest of your life. We need to attack this cancer immediately. You are not taking this seriously Aretha. You need to stop working, stop making jokes and you better buy a wig because with this drug, you'll lose your hair for sure. On your way out, go take a look at the chemo ward. It's time to pay attention Aardvark."

Half an hour later, my dad and I were standing inside the chemo ward. I walked in and my heart sank, right down to my toes. I felt like I was falling and there was no bottom. In the middle of the room was the nurses' station. They were all wearing long blue smocks, safety goggles, and gloves while handling bags of liquids. It looked like they were in a Science-Fiction movie. Along the perimeter of the room were the Patients, lying in beds with IV's hooked up to them. They were all old, with no colour in their faces or in their skin. Most of them had no hair, no eyebrows; they all looked like albinos from the movie, Powder. Their eyes were sunken in, and dazed. If I were to describe what no hope looked like, it would be this room. They had given up. The room smelled of a mixture of cleaner and coffee, like an old folk's home. Nobody was talking; there was no laughter, and no joy. The only noise I could hear was coming from the television sets. I looked up to see they were all watching a Barbara Walters' special.

Suddenly, I noticed they were all looking at my dad and me. It struck me that they must have all thought he was the one who was sick. Kids aren't supposed to get cancer before their parents. We are the ones who are supposed to take care of them. I became terrified. I didn't want to be there. My usual reaction when I feel uncomfortable is to make a joke. I immediately realized that I couldn't find the funny. There was nothing humorous about this. I didn't want to watch Barbara Walters. I ran out of the room and right into the elevator. I was so upset. For most of these people, chemotherapy was their last chance, the last bit of hope. And looking at them, how were they choosing to be inspired? They were watching Paris Hilton cry to Barbara Walters over her hair extensions. It was horrifying. It was obvious she was wearing clip-ins.

Just then, a whole bunch of people piled into the elevator and I became trapped in the back. I looked at the walls, which were plastered with signage; posters on peer support, workshops and seminars. I saw the words guilt, blame, fear. I couldn't catch my breath. The elevator stopped. The doors opened and a patient was wheeled in. He was wearing a mask and he caught me staring at him. That's when I saw the poster: "Are you afraid of dying?" That's when it hit me. I had cancer.

For three weeks, I had convinced myself that I was fine. For the last three weeks, I had been making jokes and following procedure. For the last three weeks, I had been hitting on the orderly who had reported me missing from the psych ward. Suddenly, there was so much I wanted to live for. I had just started to feel comfortable in my own skin and ready to take on the dating world. This was not part of the plan. I did not want to be known as the Cancer Girl. I didn't want to die. My mind started racing.

I found myself single with breast cancer, and spending a lot of time in the hospital. Then it hit me. I was SINGLE with BREAST CANCER and spending a lot of time in the hospital! I put it out to the universe that I wanted to meet a solid successful man and the universe responded. I was going to be meeting all sorts of successful male doctors. I was in the business of creating characters and telling stories. Why not create a character and live like that through my alter ego? From the moment the elevator doors opened again, I walked out, this time known as: The Chem-Ho.

CHAPTER 4
Becoming Chem-Ho

I've often been asked why I was so public about my battle with breast cancer; why I chose an avenue like YouTube to expose my inner demons for the whole world to see; and finally, why I would call myself a Ho!

First of all, exposing your boob woes is playing the part of Chem-Ho more effectively than online dating. Secondly, being creative is the way I deal with pain. Finally, who are you calling a Ho? Everyone has their way of dealing with trauma; some stress eat, some drink while some make bad romantic choices. I conquered the trifecta!

I deal with my pain by writing about it. I don't like to write about it directly. I prefer it as an escape. My most vivid memory was in grade four Health class. What is Health class, you would ask? This is exactly why I was trying to escape. One particular day, Mr. Andrews was giving a lecture on botulism. He was young, in his late twenties with wavy blonde hair, like Chris Atkins from The Blue Lagoon, and a matching moustache like Tom Selleck. He didn't belong in a school, but rather like he should be saving Brooke Shields from an impending coconut falling from a tree. I sat in front of the awkward girl, Linda, who was sent home weekly because she had lice. It was on that particular day that I chose to create my first character in the back of my notebook.

Her name was Jasmine and she was a spoiled rich girl from England. She was in line to be the next princess, if only she could get her shit together. She wore only one string of diamonds, which was totally frowned upon. If you want to be a proper royal, you better walk like your neck is weighing you down in jewels, like Mr.T. I was in the middle of creating Jasmine's backstory just as Mr. Andrews walked past and peered at my notebook. "Am I boring you Miss Lane?" he directed to the entire classroom. I looked at the lice girl and she sunk into the back of her chair scratching her head furiously. At that moment, he grabbed my notebook, raised it above his head and paraded to the front of the class. Visually upset, his face bore a bright shade of red while I worried his head would develop to a state where it would pop off. He sat at his desk, fuming over my lack of interest in botulism. "Don't you realize the relevance of this subject matter?" he directed, demanding an answer. I sat there dumfounded; not saying a word. He called me selfish and retarded; that I would not amount to anything. My "doodling" as he called it, was a waste of time. Doodling? I was confused because it meant something to me. I wasn't just killing time and I certainly was not retarded, that would be politically incorrect. I was creating. I was the next Harper Lee for Christ's sake. As he waved my creation back and forth, I was terrified at the notion that one of my classmates might sneak a peek mid wave and steal my ideas. Plagiarism was alive and well in elementary school.

This incident might be construed as life altering; that I would never write again, but it only fuelled the fire. It reiterated the fact that I finally knew my passion. I used my pain to create characters.

When I was first diagnosed, I knew immediately that I needed to create a character to immerse myself in. The Chem-Ho was feisty, funny, shameless, honest, fearless, and half right boob-less. I created her and she was mine. I made the videos as a way to escape so that my mind would not be occupied with negative thoughts over things

I could not control. I knew it was important to have fun and I needed it more than ever.

I made the videos for myself, but I could never have predicted their impact on others. I heard from people all over the world who said they watched as a way to heal their own reality. I started a conversation. I was able to deliver a visual timeline of the treatment process. Not only that, but I created something authentic and entertaining. I presented all of it: the tears, the uncertainty, the joy, the rejection, the anxiety, the panic, and the hot doctors on the fourth floor. Those days when the pain would be so unbearable that I could not get out of bed, I would think, "I have to get up. There are people counting on me to upload the next video, plus, I heard there is a new doctor on the fourth, I've got to check if he is single." Making the videos kept me alive. I met other women with the same prognosis as me and none of them conquered it as well as I did. Sadly, some didn't make it at all. I do have a great deal of survivor's guilt about that. I didn't even realize what survivor's guilt was until I started battling cancer. Occasionally, I felt shame about laughing, but I was making light of an otherwise dismal situation. I firmly believe laughter truly is the best medicine. I refused to believe I was going to let cancer get me down. I also refused to believe the doctor I was attempting to seduce for five months was married, and, to a man.

I'm such a firm believer in "what you think, you become" and since all I thought about was men, I became a Chem-Ho.

CHAPTER 5
Striptease

Once I finally came to terms with the fact that I have breast cancer, it caused a glitch in my life roadmap, like trying to navigate a new city and the GPS is directing in Farsi. I'm not into fads and, of course, I get the trendy cancer. I don't even like pink! I had plans to marry George Clooney, or at least date him for a weekend but watching him in re-runs of Facts of Life would have to suffice at this point. God, he was so cute in that show! No, my map was taking me on a detour at an accelerated speed for some reason. I felt I needed to reach my destination fast before I lost all of my hair and looked like Gollum from The Lord of the Rings wearing lipstick or I'd always be alone, binge-watching Tootie and Mrs. Garret try to persuade George to bend over and fix the sink.

My intense longing for a partner is nothing new. I've been on this mission a long time. And so has my mother. Every time I mention a man's name, my mother sees him as a potential husband.

"Mom, the landscapers came over today and..."

"Really, are they single?"

"Well, between the three of them they have about ten teeth and they are all wearing ankle bracelets, but I'll check."

The worst has always been the tears. Mom has one glass of wine and all of a sudden she's preparing for our guest spot on Oprah. "Oprah, I don't know why she can't find a husband. Maybe it's me, maybe I did something wrong? Maybe she could meet someone if she dressed differently?"

I don't know what she expects me to do, walk around in a wedding dress? I tried that once but I got kicked out of CrossFit. Mom has always thought I have no confidence. She once saw this episode of Oprah where a group of women were finding their inner sexiness by taking strip tease classes. So, for Christmas I got a Groupon. Thanks Mom. All this and meanwhile my dad was making payments on a Matchmaking service in my name. His account eventually went into arrears. It felt like everyone was trying to pawn me off.

I arrived at my first strip tease class to find four women huddled in a circle, clinging to their water bottles like they were life preservers. It was being held in a rented room in a seniors' complex right next door to the Kegel exercise class. A middle-aged woman turned around and smiled at me. She was wearing exercise clothes that appeared to have last been worn when Suzanne Sommers pitched The Thigh-master. Her green pants were so tight that her belly looked like a stuffed olive. She reached out to greet me. "I'm Barb. My husband left me for a twenty-year old yoga instructor. I'll show him." She accentuated her expression by raising her arms in the air to snap. "Ouch! my frigging neck."

The other ladies followed suit introducing themselves. "I'm Janice. My husband and I haven't had sex in sixteen years," she stated boldly without shame, like admitting she eats gluten.

"OH HONEY!"

We all turned around to watch an overly confident man with more femininity than Venus stride into the room like he was walking the red carpet. "You got to raise those legs in the air and pray to Jesus."

"Nobody wants to see this vagina" Janice sulked. "It looks like a cracked vase."

"OH DARLIN" he squirmed, plugging his ears. "Don't say vagina. That's so crude. Alright ladies," he clapped, "I am your STRIP instructor. I want you to choose a stripper name."

He presented a list of name tags from his man purse and placed them on the table. "This will be your name for the rest of the class, so choose a name you can really relate to. I'll start. I'm picking this one, FAIRRREEE!" He snapped his fingers and slapped his ass. The women giggled. "I love you!" Barb exclaimed reaching out to Fairy for a high five. "Don't high five," he said as he wagged his finger. I was going down the list and I found I couldn't relate to anything. Candy Cox, Venus Flytrap. Then, I found it; Merlot. I could relate to that. I drink a case a day!

After teaching us some basic moves and listening to the rattle of complaints from the ladies: "I used to be skinny and…" "Fairy, put your shirt back on," Fairy placed everyone in a line.

"Alright ladies, I want you to get down on all fours." I scanned the room and they were all doing it like he was a cult leader putting them in a trance. "Now, on the count of three, HUMP THE FLOOR." They all proceed to hump the floor like puppies in heat. As they simultaneously giggled in embarrassment, Barb reached over to high five me. My knees were sore. Fairy continued, "Don't be embarrassed ladies, you can use this in your everyday lives." Really? I imagined talking on the phone to my mother like this.

"So what are you doing tonight Ally?"

"I don't know…thought I'd stay at home and catch up on my reading, hump the floor?"

As I was pumping my pelvis up and down against the floor, everyone in class was shouting, "Go MERLOT! BE MERLOT!" I turned into Merlot faster than the Hulk turned green. I turned beat red and got brutally honest.

"Barb you've got a camel toe!" I laughed and reached over to high five her. My observation didn't receive the response I had hoped for. My Groupon didn't get used up and to this day, I can't look at the floor without cringing, but I did get a punch card for "Kegel for seniors." So, the strip classes were a bust. My mother was at a loss and had resorted to persuading my friends to give me dating advice.

First, there is my friend Sue, the teacher. Sue is one of those people that will read an article about something and all of a sudden she is an expert. She devoured a Dr. Phil book and believed she had transformed into the T.V. psychologist. She even talked with a Texan droll.

"You know what your problem is? You're desperate for love, you're never going to find love unless you love yourself." My response was not what she was expecting. "I have three broken vibrators, overdue charges at the adult video store and a massaging shower-head I have to replace weekly. Loving myself is not the problem." "You go to an adult video store?" she retorted, fixing her Don't Mess with Texas belt buckle.

Then there's my friend Jessica. She got married right out of high school, has three kids, and has never had to date. "I know what your problem is, you're clueless. That guy over there has been staring at you for half an hour, now go talk to him."

"He's 12." I respond sharply.

"No he isn't."

"There's a sign above his head that says Happy 12th Birthday. I used to babysit for his mom." I don't know what sort of available men Jessica thought she could find me at Chuckie Cheese.

We all have questions in life that make us uncomfortable. Why are you single? Why don't you have kids? Then you have a kid and the next question is: When are you having another? Then the next question: When is your kid moving out? All of these questions before your second trimester is even over. It's hard to give an answer that satisfies most people, especially when you don't know the answer either. My retort is often: Why does your husband wear pleated pants? The only difference is that I truly want to know. The real answer is I don't know why I'm STILL single. I also don't know why I watch Teen Moms, but I do.

I believe in the expression: The sexiest body part of a woman is confidence. Although my mom believes I had lost mine, it wasn't always so. Ever since the day I discovered acting, I believed I could accomplish anything. Acting is an illusion of taking oneself and transporting them into the character. It is very freeing. I am happier when I am performing. I feel indestructible. My biggest wish is that the Dramatic Arts become mandatory in the school system. My other wish is that grown men stop wearing Crocs.

If students had Arts in their lives, it would solve so many problems. Young girls would stop starving themselves and insulting each other. Young boys would stop bullying. In high school, my nicknames were 'Thunder thighs' and 'Bubble Butt'. My butt was so ahead of its time. I'm an innovator. The Kardashians owe me a royalty payment. Those names didn't bother me though as I never really focused on the way I looked. If I had, I wouldn't have chosen to sport a purple Mohawk and wear our basement curtains as a skirt. I had other things to do. That all changed when I turned 27. I fell in love with a very attractive motocross rider.

He was very fit with the deepest hazel eyes, beautiful white teeth, with a smile that wouldn't quit. He was traditionally handsome with chiselled features but he dressed in a laid-back snowboarder style, which I found irresistible. His name was Jody and he introduced me to the world of extreme sports. Through his encouragement, I learned how to ride a motorcycle and a mountain bike, through terrain saved for wild animals. Our relationship was fun and thrilling. He would always remind me that I was not like other girls. I was refreshing and real. I instantly gravitated towards his friends and I spent every waking hour at his house. It was the relationship of my dreams: hot boyfriend, thrilling adventures, and a new set of fun friends.

When the summer ended and before the snow began to fall, Jody grew more and more distant. He was spending time with a group of people he normally would have considered 'plastic'; frequenting nightclubs, talking about money, and his behaviour became controlling. Then, out of the blue, he looked at me point blank and said, "I'm not attracted to you anymore." I was dumbfounded. My body felt like it was in free-fall, like driving down a steep hill. Only the hill didn't end, stabbing me with the insults, picking my body apart from head to toe.

At the end of his Simon Cowell critique, the shock of his words had diminished and I was left with the realization that I would not be moving onto the next round. In the span of ten minutes, I went from being a healthy, confident, and unstoppable woman to a fat, unattractive and unlovable loser. Words cut deep. To add insult to injury, a week later, he began dating someone he used to tell me to "never be like" as she wore so much make up she could make a drag queen squirm. It didn't matter that I had my own life, passion and dreams, all that mattered was the size of my butt and it was, to quote Jody, embarrassing. This was news to me. I thought embarrassment was defined as listening to Nickleback. I realized that being real and authentic meant nothing. I suddenly understood that all that men wanted were pretty, skinny girls. Looking at myself in the mirror translated to humiliation and I had to do something about it.

The first thing I did was run to the hairdresser and requested a Meg Ryan haircut. Jody told me Meg is what all men are attracted to. When I arrived home from the salon showcasing a new hairdo, my roommate asked, "Why did you cut your hair like my mom?"

The next step on the roadmap of life was becoming transfixed with women's bodies. I didn't like the person I had become but I couldn't control my emotions. Anger and jealously had possessed me. I hated all thin women. Why were they blessed with long legs and tiny hips? Why was I given magnified curves and fat knees? It was a struggle to look at myself in the mirror. Every day was a struggle to feel worthy.

It thus sparked an endless cycle of dieting and self-hate. Exercise was never an issue for me. I had always been consistent and enjoyed all sorts of outdoor activities. Nope, if I wanted attention from the opposite sex, I had to lose weight. I started with my diet. I thought I ate fairly well. I have been a vegetarian most of my life and fast food does not appeal to me. Even though I thought I was doing everything right, the man I loved, didn't love me anymore because I was "too fat to be seen in public with."

For the next seven years I struggled, always perusing the grocery store and buying anything in a package marked 'diet,' 'low fat', 'low calorie,' and 'free'. I became a diet food junkie. No, scrap that. I became a 'diet' junkie. Bouncing from one diet to the next, hoping for the miracle cure that would transform me into the ideal woman. I made food choices based on calories, not nutrition. Why eat a nutrient rich avocado when I could have a bag of candy for the same amount of calories? One day after devouring an entire bag of sugar free chocolate peanut butter cups, I hopped on my motorcycle. Five minutes later, I found myself lying on the side of the road, in a ditch, curled up in a ball, with the most immense stomach pains. Delusional, I had convinced myself that I had the flu even though on the chocolate bar, in bright orange letters the package read 'WARNING, MAY CAUSE ANAL LEAKAGE'. Leakage? This was more like a rear end ejaculation. I had to wear a maxi pad on my ass. I was in an aspartame fog that I couldn't navigate my way out of. Addicted to diet foods, my body wasn't receiving any nutrients except for the occasional post-hangover banana. The way I felt about myself transcended in the way I treated it.

So when my mother proclaimed I had no confidence, I guess she was right, even though she believes she is ALWAYS right. Last week when I asked her to google a recipe, she said, "Google is wrong." This coming from a woman who thinks googling is a rapid way to whisk eggs.

So where did those years of self-hatred get me? Was living on a diet of processed packaged diet foods the answer to my self-worth? I was in the same place I was, seven years previous although. now I owned family sized packages of adult diapers. I couldn't wait another seven years to get my life together. I had to take care of my body and my heart. Chemotherapy was going to be hard on me physically so I had to treat it right. No more diet foods, no more alcohol binges instigated by anger over not losing weight from the diet foods, no more self-hatred. NO MORE! I was ready and there was no stopping me, except for that damn IV attached to my arm, although I found it made a nice accessory, like a purse or a cane.

The Chem-Ho had a mission. Not only to meet a man, but to meet a man worthy of me.

CHAPTER 6
The Wig out Party

Cancer is a great excuse to throw a party. I don't know how many times in my life I have tried to organize a party and nobody shows up, so I end up making out with the only available single man in the room. As soon as you mention, cancer, EVERYBODY shows up. I knew my life was about to change. So I decided the best thing to do about the cards I was dealt, was to throw a party. If I was going to lose my hair and have to wear wigs then all of my friends were wearing wigs too. I decided to call it "The Wig out Party".

Two days before my first chemo treatment, almost a hundred people showed up to my five hundred square foot condo, each wearing a wig. People got right into character with their wigs, and right into the 7-layer Mexican bean dip. The toilet got clogged twice. All I can say is men look hot in mullets! Let's face it, who isn't attracted to Joe Dirt? I was overwhelmed with the amount of love that was in that room, and the amount of bodily gases.

Friends came that I had not spoken to in years. Ex-boyfriends came that I had not slept with in years. I had no idea how many friends I actually had. I also had no idea how many men I had slept with. Maybe it wasn't a good idea to line them up like that.

There was one guy in particular that I was very excited to see in my house. His name was Scott and he was a stand-up comedian who I had befriended over the past few months. He walked in the door with large black wings strapped to his back and said, "I thought that invitation said it was a wing party?" I didn't know if it was a joke, or if he couldn't read, but either way, he made me laugh.

I had a huge crush on him and I knew that if he were in my house, it would only be a matter of time and a matter of Merlot before he would be in my bed. Normally I would wait at least one date before I made my move, but I was on a time crunch. In a few days' time, I would be strapped to an IV pole, so it was now or never. I made several attempts to get a moment alone with him, but the only room that wasn't occupied with people was my pantry. I tried an impromptu game of Two Minutes in the Closet, but everyone just shook their heads thinking: "she's drunk." Well duh…I have cancer! Now take your shirt off!

My friend Alice was also flirting with him heavy. He told her she had a nice singing voice. Ok, this was a HUGE mistake. It is true, Alice has a very nice singing voice but instead of joining a band or choir, or even frequenting karaoke nights, she would break out into A-cappella in the most inappropriate places. For example she sang Helen Reddy's "I am Woman" while passing by a trans-genders equal rights rally. Her habit became quite an embarrassment amongst our group of friends, especially when she would expect us to do actions. I knew that if she kept up her flirting and singing, neither one of us was getting any action, and if she got my party doing the wave, I was shutting the whole thing down.

I pulled her aside and told her that I liked Scott. She was a little upset but understood. After all, I had the cancer card. She then tried to end the conversation with an Air Supply medley. I left her singing "All by myself" by herself.

At this time Scott had struck up a conversation with John. John was a musician I knew through my comedy nights. I hosted a comedy night every Sunday at a local bar and he was one of the regular patrons. Each time I saw John, he was always laughing at my jokes, so I instantly liked him. It didn't matter that he was always drunk. He brought his guitar, a bottle of Schnapps and his cheerful John Candy like oaf of a friend Steve.

As the night wore on, I had four glasses of wine going simultaneously and ten different conversations. John and I polished off his bottle by having a shooter contest. I thought he looked rather cute in his dread lock wig…or maybe it wasn't a wig. It didn't matter.

My vision was blurry and somehow I had forgotten how to walk. I was slurring my words and I think I may have barfed inside my mouth but I decided it was all in the name of training for chemo. Also, when you have cancer, people don't seem to mind if you get highly intoxicated and slap their husband's ass. They actually encourage it. So as Scott and John were in my office jamming to "We Will Rock You," I was laying them on every ass in the room. After I washed my hands and came into the office to go in for the kill, there was Alice singing the first act of "A Chorus Line". During the line "God I hope I get it," I was praying she was singing about contracting syphilis.

I spent the rest of that night in the room sitting between Scott and John, singing and slapping. What I didn't realize is how similar the two looked. Maybe it was the fact that they kept trading clothes or that my eyes were completely crossed.

As the party started to wind down, I found myself alone for the first time with Scott. It was time to make my move. I looked around to see if Alice was in my sights but found out that she had gone to the neighbours after someone told her he had Rock Band. Scott and I were only chatting for a few moments when he said something so profound:

"I saw you have a huge bed."

"Yes," I answered.

"Can I share it with you?"

"EVERYBODY OOOOUUUUUUTTTTTTTTT!"

Scott immediately went downstairs and waited for me in my bedroom. It took me about ten minutes to kick the rest of the people out of my house. People can turn into crying babies when you tell them the party is over, especially when you pour their drinks down the drain. I didn't care. I was getting laid two days before chemo. When everyone left I looked around my empty condo and saw the remnants of a successful party. I thought to myself: You are loved Allison. Look around. Look at how much wine is left. You are so loved.

I took a deep breath. The sole survivor was Steve, the John Candy look alike. He looked just like Uncle Buck, passed out on the couch with a pink ladies wig on and my dog Peggy licking the 7-layer dip off his face. I put a blanket over him, took the beer out of his hand and turned the lights off. I grabbed a glass of wine and a condom out of the fridge and ran downstairs. Yes, I keep my condoms in the fridge. I heard they last longer.

When I got into my room, the lights were already out and I slid into bed right next to Scott with my wig still on. He pressed up against me and immediately started kissing my neck. He smelled of booze, cigarettes, and 7-Layer dip. It was all very romantic.

"Take that wig off," he whispered, "I like you just the way you are." I had my long blonde hair cut short to prepare me for the drastic change. I was very self-conscious about the short cut but he put me right at ease. I reached down under the covers and something else was definitely NOT at ease.

We got right down to business and it was better than I ever expected it to be. I closed my eyes and saw the beginning of our life together: our wedding at Hooters, the archway made out of beer cans we drunk the night before, my dog as the ring bearer, my dad wearing a belt, Mom writing an invoice for the beer...

He pulled me closer and gently ran his fingers over my skin and through my hair. I shared in his excitement and could tell that he was close.

"Scott I can't believe this is happening," I gushed, "I've liked you for so long."

He took a big breath and stopped moving. He looked at me almost dumbfounded. Had he not known how I had felt? This must have been a total boost to his ego. The life of the party had liked him and ONLY him. I was awaiting a mutual response. I got the guy I wanted and it was totally worth it. I could finally breathe knowing that the next six months were going to be alright. I didn't have to worry any longer. I wasn't going to go through this alone; he could take me to the cancer centre, hold my head as I puked, and shave his initials into my head. Everything was going to be okay because I now had a man by my side.

"I'm not Scott," he answered.

My heart started pounding as I flashed back to an hour or so earlier. Scott and John played a joke on me and traded clothes and wigs. I quickly pieced together that the man I invited into my bed was John, not Scott. It was an unfortunate accident, like the week before when I mistook a fat woman for a pregnant one and tried to listen to her belly. They had not changed back and I was sleeping with the wrong person.

"I knew that," I giggled. I was mortified, and he finished what he started.

I felt so sorry for John and didn't want to let him in on my secret that I actually tried to date him afterwards. It didn't last long; he was an imposter.

CHAPTER 7
Door #3

To begin my breast cancer journey, I had my first date with the surgeon, or I guess it's called an appointment? I was going to be expected to make a decision regarding the outcome of my breasts: to keep them or not to keep them? This was the Chem-Ho's first appearance and the only decision I was concerned about was: cleavage or no cleavage?

My mother decided to come along as my wing-man and booked the next flight out. When the booking agent Barb asked if she had a frequent flyer card she replied: "My daughter has CANCER," and then her and Barb spent the next two hours crying together. Barb was a mother too with a young daughter, so they had a lot to talk about. And Mom had a lot of coupons to claim. My mother hung up the phone after receiving a complimentary one-way flight and an invite to Barb's daughter's graduation. She was ecstatic.

On our way to my blind date meeting spot, my mother managed to let the train station attendant, the Safeway bagger, and the busker playing for loose change in on the fact that her daughter had CANCER. From that moment my friends no longer referred to me in conversations as: "You know my friend Ally, the blonde one?" or "The single one?" Now I was known as: "The one with the CANCER."

Right after my diagnosis, I went to a neighbourhood block party with my neighbour Shari, who thought I could use some cheering up. From the onset of introductions, Shari let the neighbourhood know: "Ally has CANCER." All of a sudden I received the pity stares, the first helping of potato salad and my wine glass was constantly topped up. I drank so much that I fell asleep in the condo president's rose bush. I woke up to her husband fertilizing my backside. When I stumbled onto their lawn with my hands down my pants pulling out thorns, the wife, smacking her gum with a face full of make-up shook her head and said in a thick Italian accent: "Poor thing has cancer...go to the store and get her some more red wine," handing him a twenty. I was starting to realize that CANCER had its advantages. I didn't have to wait in line, I was never put on hold, and I had a house full of Merlot.

I didn't mind the attention. It felt good to get off on a speeding ticket because I was wearing a head scarf and get my coffee card stamped up when all I wanted was to use the washroom.

When Mom and I entered the surgeon's office, we had to walk through the waiting area to get to the reception desk. The room was empty except for the stacks of magazines that filled the chairs. The room looked like it belonged in an episode of Hoarders. This was great! Maybe if he couldn't get rid of old magazines then maybe he wouldn't let me part with my boob. I may not have to make this decision after all. I introduced myself to the receptionist who was fuelling calls with a switchboard ringing off the hook like it was the voting line on American Idol. "I'm here to meet THE SURGEON, let's hope he's single. Too much cleavage?" She looked confused. I looked down at my chest and realized I had some remnants of my lunch in between my boobs. "Hope he likes KFC," I laughed nervously. Mom interjected by tapping her hand on the desk. "She has CANCER...is this the new issue of Oprah?" My mom leaned in and whispered, "I'm taking it home. They are almost six dollars at the drug store." The receptionist was not amused. "You'll be one of his last patients, he retires next month. Have a seat." I was very disappointed. I wore a push-up bra for an old guy?

This potential suitor did not meet my #1 MUST HAVE. I followed the advice of Patti Stenger, The Millionaire Matchmaker. Her "go to" recommendation for meeting the love of your life is to keep a list of your 5 MUST HAVES. If they don't meet all five on your list, MOVE ON.

The first must have on my list is firm testicles. It's not to say old men have saggy balls but I didn't want to find out. Not my cup of tea, I'm not into tea bagging. I turned around to face the waiting area and caught my mother stuffing Martha Stewart Living into her purse. I picked up the latest issue of Shape with Sheryl Crow on the cover. She was in her forties in a string bikini and I thought: "She is gorgeous and she had breast cancer, and her boobs are still hers." I flipped to read the article while Mom was cutting out a recipe for lentil salad. Sheryl had had a lumpectomy and went through radiation treatment. She spoke of receiving treatment in the morning and going out every afternoon to ride her horses. She changed her diet to be completely organic and began a cleaner, healthier lifestyle. I thought about it and it didn't seem bad at all. If

Sheryl was able to keep her boobs and ride horses, I could keep my boobs and ride cowboys. It made sense, right?

The next magazine featured Christina Applegate on the cover. She had a double mastectomy and already had a new set of C cups nestled into her size two frame. She said her new boobs looked really good and her boyfriend loved them. I thought, "Okay, maybe a new set of boobs would help me meet a man?" She had the operation and was back on the set of her television show within a month. Christina had chosen the operation that removed the breasts so that she didn't require any other treatment PLUS she received a brand new rack to boot! I thought that didn't seem so bad either. New boobs, new boyfriend, no problem!

When the receptionist called my name, I walked into the appointment confident that no matter what the surgeon's decision, I would be over this within a month and have a cowboy to bring home for Christmas.

My surgeon was an older gentleman with white hair and a heavy droll. He looked like Kenny Rogers in scrubs, minus the Botox. He actually wasn't half bad. No Ally, he has old balls. He got right to it. "Let's take a look at your breasts." That is the great thing about having boob cancer; everybody wants to take a look. I was getting to second base with every doctor in town and I didn't even have to slip him a Roofie, or tell his wife.

Old Balls proceeded to deliver his findings: a quarter sized tumour and two French fries from my snack pack. "In terms of the surgery, you have a few options. I can remove both breasts, one breast, OR you can keep your breasts, but in that case you will have to endure chemotherapy and radiation. So, what do you want to do?"

I felt like I was in an episode of Let's Make a Deal. Did I want what was behind Door #1? Then it came to me. There was so much my boobs hadn't done yet. I had not been the recipient of a motorboat, gone for a proper bra fitting or flashed my titties at a hockey game, although, I did show a nipple once for a large double-double, and a Timbit.

I came to the realization that I'd been taking my breasts for granted. I treated my breasts like blobs of fat, but not anymore. My boobs were mine and I was going to be proud of them. I would cart them around like trophies. I would welcome anyone to touch them, squeeze them, fondle them, and poke them. My boobs would be public boobs. Could you imagine if I had cancer of the clitoris? Never mind, no one would be able to find it. So I decided to keep my boobs. And, if I was going to go through hell to save them, then I was going to show them off.

I took in a deep breath, relieved that I would not become Uni-boob. "I want door #3."

"If you do that, then you'll have to get radiation," he stressed.

"Done," I said.

My mother, whom I had forgotten was here peeked her head around the corner. "Is she making the right decision?" she asked with her arms full of sample birth control packs. I waved my arms at her dismissing her from the room. I didn't want to hear his answer. I didn't want to lose my boob; right decision or not, I wasn't prepared to let them go. I was also not prepared to know what my mother was going to do with a year's supply of Tri-Phasal.

"It's a good decision," he responded looking at her confused, as she tried to steal some of his prescription pads. "If we remove the breast entirely she will not require further treatment, but with the lumpectomy, she will." I would take the Sheryl Crow route. It was the easiest decision of my life. After feeling so scared that I would have to lose my breasts, at that moment I felt a huge sense of relief. With breasts, I would still have the chance to find a man. I would also be able to safe more leftovers in my cleavage. It was a win-win.

CHAPTER 8
The Top Ten Things NOT to say to someone with Cancer

Even though I made the decision to keep my breasts and go through radiation and chemotherapy, I am the Chem-Ho for a reason; I don't think I was prepared for what I was going to have to endure. The pity-guilt comments and acts of kindness from others had begun before treatment but now that I was actually going through it, the "I can totally relate to what you're going through" and the "I know just what to say to make you feel better" stories had begun. Going through radiation was hard work and I didn't have the patience to deal with everyone else's bullshit, so pardon me if I sound bitter when recounting what I remember.

1. "I wouldn't get chemo if I were you. Have you tried an organic diet and putting hot rocks on your stomach?"

   Yes, and after I'm done, I'm going to steal the eggs from your free range and throw them at your Off The Grid Tiny House. You're not a doctor, you're my mailman. Look, I'm Canadian and we happen to be blessed with a health care system where we don't have to pay for cancer treatment. So, if I can get chemo, I'm getting chemo! Plus, the guy that collects the garbage in the chemo ward is really hot and the nurses tell me he is as dumb as a stump, so I can't lose!

2. "You have cancer. I know how you feel… I have a hangnail."

   Don't compare your paper-cuts, your bad periods, or the annoying receptionist at your work to what I'm going through! Believe me; at this point, I would trade anything to get a bad period than go through this.

3. "You should meet my cousin's next door neighbour's sister's friend's aunt from a previous marriage once removed. She had cancer, you should talk."

Yah, we should talk. Does she like chocolate too? If so, that would be freaky. We'd be like, soul mate sisters…once removed. Listen folks, forty percent of all people get cancer in their lifetime. It's not rare. What's rare is finding a man who cleans up his toenails clippings and only pees in the toilet. Now that's rare.

4. "I want to be there for you but I'm scared."

You're scared? You've got a hair coming out of that mole longer than the drive through lane at Tim Hortons. I'm the one who should be scared. Cancer isn't airborne. You're not going to catch it by talking to me. My boobs aren't going to fall off right in front of you…but that mole of yours might.

5. "I've been such a good friend to you. You need me."

No…what I need is a case of wine and a Costco size chocolate bar. When you go through something traumatic in your life, you really find out who your friends are. True friends don't make it about themselves. They bring you endless bottles of red.

6. "Are you still alive? Call me if you're dead."

This was an actual phone message I received from my sister. She always knows the right thing to say.

7. "Stop pulling the cancer card."

Well, you keep pulling out your Starbuck's card and I don't complain about that. At The Tom Baker Cancer Centre, they give patients an actual cancer card. At the height of my treatments, I was going to the centre up to five times a week, and I had had to show my card every time I went. So SORRY if I keep pulling it out, but they keep asking for it. What do you want me to do?

8. "Does this mean you can't work because I am looking for a new job?"

Now because I own my own business, people thought I wouldn't be able to run it. I had a regular gig hosting a comedy night. Don't phone me asking if you can take my spot without asking if I'm out of wine. Wait...Am I an alcoholic? Oh who cares, I have cancer!

9. "You're so skinny! You look great."

Yes, please! Tell me I look great because everyone loves a compliment. It's a lot of work putting on false eyelashes, drawing in eyebrows, and maintaining a wig, but the real reason I've lost weight is because I'm puking non-stop. My mouth sores are so bad that it feels like Tobasco sauce on an open wound. Anything with flavour that I eat stings my tongue. I'm shitting all the time. I've got haemorrhoids the size of golf balls and when I try to shit it feels like razor blades being passed through my asshole. I have horrible acid reflux and it feels like something is stuck in my throat. So all in all, it's just better that I don't eat, which is another reason why I'm so skinny! I don't understand why society looks up to celebrities who are being led around by their hipbones. They have no diet secrets. That's bullshit. They are not doing yoga and living off of a macrobiotic diet. They are not eating, plain and simple. Yoga is hard people! When I was sick, there was no way I could hold a downward dog unless I was holding onto the toilet. So, please don't tell me the reason why I look great is because I'm skinny. I'm skinny because I'm not eating. That is a reason for concern, NOT for celebration. Throw me a party and feed me cake through a tube. I'm hungry goddammit and this isn't a choice, no matter how good I look in low-rise jeans.

10. "You gained your weight back, that's too bad."

    What's too bad is when your boyfriend hasn't gone down on you in two years, that's too bad. I'm sorry I'm such a big disappointment because I'm finally strong enough to lift something heavier than your personality. I'm a mountain girl who likes to ski, eat carbs, and has booty larger than a thumbtack. Hallelujah!

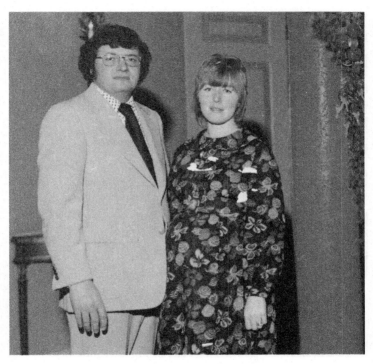

Mom and Dad, 4 days prior to
my birth. Yep, I'm in there.

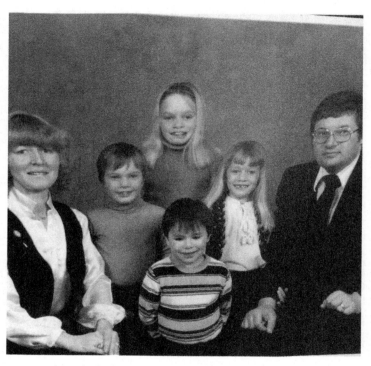

The whole family. I'm pictured far right next to
my Dad, wearing miniature clogs as jewelry?

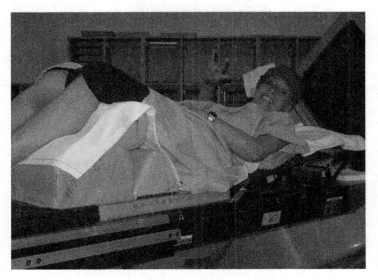

Getting ready for radiation.

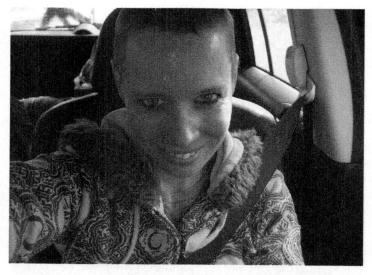

Hair is starting to grow back. In 2009, I
embarked on a North American road trip
with my dog in between rounds of treatments.
This photo is taken in San Francisco.

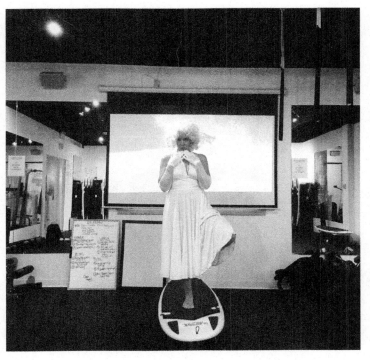

Combining my two passions, acting and surfing. I showed up at the Surfset Fitness studio en route to a Marilyn Monroe gig.

CHAPTER 9
Loyalty and the Leather Jacket

Attempting to drink a shooter with two broken hands is an art form. Luckily, I have the cute-looking Latin guy to help me. Latin men are my type. "I look Latin because I AM Latin," he retorts, gargling a Sambuca. He tells me he is a florist, which clearly translates to: he likes his snapdragons hard. Note to self- ''Add new MUST HAVE- Heterosexual." He does meet a lot of criteria on my list. Top of my list: LOYAL. The florist is that. He keeps checking in on me, ensuring I am doing all right. I must look pathetic, with casts up to my elbows, sulking at the wood, bobbing for bar nuts. I learned about loyalty the hard way.

Ally Lane

My friend Sue was always there for me. She was a transplant to Calgary, single, and ran a small business out of her home. We would talk on the phone every day for hours, exchanging stories of difficulties we had as female entrepreneurs. We were comrades and allies of sorts, dishing out advice, and giving support when needed.

I had not seen Sue for a few days when she arrived at my doorstep looking radiant. She appeared to be a completely different person, alive and glowing. The stress that usually occupied her face was gone and she looked younger, thinner and happier.

"What happened to you?" I admired.

"I went on a personal development weekend retreat," she gloated.

This retreat had changed her, it had removed the baggage she was carrying around and left her refreshed, with a new outlook on life.

"Give me some of that!" I begged in jest.

"I have a coupon for five hundred dollars off, it's yours," she teased.

A week later, I entered a dark and dusty conference room set in the industrial area of the city. I arrived seeking all the answers for my singledom, hoping to be given the tools to assist me in finding the man of my dreams.

The room was full; fifty plus people occupied the space all seeking answers for their life's woes. The teacher, Lynn, was an attractive blond woman in her forties, who commanded the room with her overly confident presence.

"These are the rules; no drinking for five days; no caffeine; no talking about the program and if you leave the room you cannot come back."

Did I sign up for Fight Club? Where is Meatloaf and his manly boobs? I scanned the room. The only likeness I found was a fat man staring at MY boobs.

The room was set up conference style with rows of chairs all facing the podium. At the front, a bare stage with a stool, a microphone and stand just like an intimate Jerry Seinfeld concert, only more expensive! Lynn welcomed the stage as an open forum, to address our experiences. "Hell yeah!" I thought. Nothing excites an actor more than an open stage. My mind started racing with new material I wanted to share. "My vibrator jokes will kill," I chuckled to myself. I was itching to be the first to share, showing the rest how to command a crowd. I would be a hit!

"Take a look around the room," Lynn instructed.

I perused the room and looked for any young single man in a vulnerable state. The only thing I noticed was the fat man staring at me. I did a double take and realized he had a lazy eye.

"Remember where you are sitting," she continued.

Of course I'd remember. I was too far from the stage.

"We're all going to work together to remove the chairs and place them at the side of the room. I want you to do it in less than a minute and I'm timing it. GO!"

At that moment, it was anarchy. We rushed around the room in complete chaos as she blasted the score from Star Wars over the loudspeaker. Men were sweating, women were crying and the fat man's lazy eye went straight.

"Good. Now you have thirty-seconds to put them back. GO".

At the end of the exercise she requested a volunteer come up and speak into the microphone. I was too busy smelling my armpits and missed my first chance.

A woman approached the microphone.

"How did that exercise make you feel?" Lynn asked.

"I felt panicked."

"Why?" she continued.

"There was a lot of pressure to do well."

"Why?" Lynn repeated.

"I felt I had to do well."

Lynn repeated the words WHY over and over again, prodding the answer out of her until exhaustion. Then she spoke, "I was molested when I was three!"

The entire room gasped. I sunk into my chair.

For five days, I heard some tragic stories. I felt for the people in real pain. I listened to heart wrenching journeys. I realized that being a single woman was so trivial. I was embarrassed about my objectives for the week. These people had real problems. I never spoke up. I never shared. I vowed to never go up and speak into that microphone. I just sat back and listened.

I never received any dating tips, but what I learned was much more valuable. I was so busy trying to be heard, that I never took the time to listen to people. I knew part of it stemmed from a childhood of being ignored. With a family in chaos, I never wanted to create any problems for my parents so I just tried to survive. As an adult I tried to make up for lost time and as a result I was always the loudest, most obnoxious person in the room. Yep, I was the annoying girl. So I guess I did learn some great dating advice. I need to listen. Not only listen to potential suitors but listen to my instincts. A few months later, I met the Ass Man and I did a lot of listening. I listened to him talk about his butt, his butt career, and how everybody loved his butt. Yes, it's true. Everybody loves an ass.

As for Sue, she stayed in my life up until my cancer diagnosis. She dropped off a bag of wheat germ and blueberries on my doorstep and I never heard from her again. I was devastated over it and not a day goes by that I don't think about what caused her to exonerate the friendship. I received no explanation for her actions. All I got was silence and a lot of diarrhoea. Wheat germ, really?

I understand it is hard to figure out what to do for someone, or what to say to them when they are diagnosed with an illness. When you go through something as difficult as cancer, you truly learn who your friends are.

In the first few days of my diagnosis, I conducted the rounds of phone calls to my friends. One of the first people I called was my friend Lara. She is a person I greatly admire. I have never seen her lose control. She takes life in stride. Her life is calm and devoid of tragedy. Why? Simple, she creates a calm life devoid of tragedy. Both her son and her husband are very laid back and relaxed. When I am around her family, they instantly create serenity. But when my family is around, they immediately create gastro-intestinal issues. I knew that when I called Lara, she would enlighten me with her wisdom.

"Lara. Are you sitting down? I have something to tell you. It's not good news. Don't be afraid. I'm going to try to tell you this without crying."

"Jeez, what is it?" she asked.

"I can't believe I am about to say this."

"Oh my god! What is it?"

"I…I," my voice was shaking. "I have breast cancer" I declared.

There was a long pause and I imagined her crying on the other end. Then I heard her take a deep breath and she spoke, "SO?"

"What?" I answered dumbfounded.

"That's it? That's all it is? You're lucky. You can join a dragon boat team," she joked.

Now, some may interpret her reaction as insensitive, but I know Lara. I know what she meant. She knew I could spin it into something positive. I was not joining a bloody dragon boat team but I was seeking to ride something long and fast, so she was on the right track. Bad dirty joke, but what do you expect? My name is Ally Lane. My name is from English stock and it literally means where you are from. So I'm from a back alley. The Brits couldn't be more direct. If my dirty jokes offend you don't blame me. Blame my roots. Talk about loyalty, she was there for my first chemo treatment, and now she's wiping my ass because I have two broken hands.

There were a lot of lovely gestures sent my way throughout my illness. Every morning, I woke up to a new care package on my doorstep. People really know what a chemo patient wants to help them feel better: anything pink! What did people expect me to do with 48 pink journals and 75 pink boas? Should I write my suicide note and choke myself? Give me something pink I can use, like Pepto-Bismol.

My chemo treatments were three weeks apart of which the first two weeks I spent lying on the bathroom floor. I knew the chemo would make me barf and quite frankly, my ass could use a little shrinking, so I was kind of looking forward to the weight loss without the effort. I didn't realize how sick it would make me. At first, it was all very punk rock. The vomiting, the swearing, and when

I barfed all over my CBGB's t-shirt, I knew I was cool enough to be invited to Keith Richard's next cocktail party. One day I'd step on the scale and I would be ten pounds lighter and the next day I could be ten pounds heavier. It made it very difficult to decide what to wear on a Friday night. The one side effect I was not prepared for and could not see any benefits to, was the extreme constipation. It wasn't the bloating that bothered me; I have done that many times myself after too much diet coke. After the screaming and the pushing, I developed the worst case of haemorrhoids my nurse had ever seen. It was like a giant golf ball hanging off my backside. I think I could hear it talking to me. Nothing says sexy like a girl bringing an inflatable donut as a seat cushion on a date.

The barfing and the golf ball finally subsided three days before my next treatment. I had three days of cramming in every little piece of adventure I could before I was back in the bathroom, crawled up in a ball, with an ice cube shoved down my pants.

This actually happened once when my temperature went over 38 degrees, I had a white blood count of zero, and my body had infections in every open orifice. I was rushed to the hospital and had to spend six days getting pumped up with morphine and a blood transfusion, watching a weekend marathon of Judge Judy in Spanish. The only saving grace was the parade of very hot young doctors making their rounds every evening. I was like a contestant on The Bachelorette, "this episode sponsored by Preparation H." I had always used it for the bags under my eyes, so now I had one tube for my eyes and the other for my butt. It wasn't until I got them mixed up that I had to start labeling them.

So here I was, three days before my next treatment and ten pounds lighter, sans inflatable donut. I was able to walk around without limping. So when my friend Kristi called to go out for happy hour drinks with two of her male friends, Ben and Mike, I jumped at the chance.

As soon as I heard Mike's name, I applied a fresh coat of Prep H, put on my bleach blond Pamela Anderson wig, my hot little leather jacket that I bought a size too small, saving for the day I could fit into it, and praise the lord, that day had come.

Mike was a local director in town and I had auditioned for him before. He was somewhat of a legend in the film community and I was excited about the opportunity. I had always had a crush on him from the first time I saw his big brown dopey bloodshot eyes. He was casting for two parts. The first was described as: "The gorgeous sexy lead that looks like she just stepped out of an American Apparel ad." I did not feel gorgeous or sexy. My idea of sex appeal was farting in bed. The other role was for her "mascot". I knew I would be a shoe in for the mascot. I actually worked as one while I was a university student studying theatre. Imagine my surprise when I was offered the part of the sexy lead. From that day on, I was smitten.

Now, Kristi had a crush on Ben. She had let him know by sleeping with him a few days before. This wasn't new for her. In the year that I had known her, she had crushed on every guy she had had a conversation with, including the door-to-door salesman asking her to switch cable companies. Kristi also had this narcissistic notion that every guy she talked to was in love with her. In her opinion, if her conversation lasted longer than a burp, the man was deeply infatuated, and she was filing for a restraining order. I couldn't help but wonder if Ben was any different. Their rendezvous happened after a drunken evening. She called me the next morning to tell me the news. I was busy barfing and wasn't in the mood for the weekly play-by-play of her latest conquest.

I told her I was sick and her response was, "Oh! ok...I'll hold."

She told me in detail about how they ran into each other at a martini bar, the number of drinks every person in the bar drank, and how they ended the night in her futon. The next morning Ben awoke to the sound of Kristi analyzing their evening together. She came to the conclusion that "they should have just stayed friends". She could have been picked up by Brad Pitt and whisked off in a jet but she'd still need to analyze and talk it to death. And men LOVE to talk about their feelings, right?

When I arrived at the pub, the three of them were already sitting on the patio. Kristina was sitting next to Ben; already looking extremely bored, obviously awaiting my arrival so she could give her analysis of the evening thus far. Quite frankly, I didn't care. I had three days to get some sort of action before I was in the literal "pooper". There was an empty seat next to Mike, who looked as dopey as ever. Tonight, I was making my move. There would, of course, be some minor details to work out. First of all, I still didn't know how I was going to keep my eyebrows, eyelashes and wig on during the act.

As soon as I sat down, Kristi eyed me up and down like I was a rival contestant on The Bachelor.

"That jacket is trouble."

Trouble? It wasn't even real leather! I didn't hand sew it out of baby seals for god sakes. I think it was her way of paying me a compliment because she saw the way the boy's eyes lit up when I approached the table. I was so happy to be out of the house, feeling good and out on the town. A smile goes a long way people. Remember that!

As soon as I sat down, Ben leaned in very excited. "How are you feeling?"

"Today I feel great, so tonight I want to parrrtayy!" I said winking at Mike.

I had no time to be subtle.

Ben continued, "I've been watching all of your videos. They're so good and very touching; you made me cry."

Kristi did not look impressed. Apparently if anyone is going to make her new man cry, it should be her.

Ben kept dishing out the compliments, "She is so brave. Have you seen them?"

Mike just nodded his head. I was quite relieved. I didn't want him to know I was keeping my options open. In my last video, I hit on the garbage boy at the hospital and chased after him with my IV still intact.

I was so excited to chat with Mike. Unfortunately Ben was pretty excited too. He kept asking me question after question. He was a great conversationalist and I could see why Kristi liked him, but come on, enough about me already! The table talk became Ben and I engrossed in conversation while Kristi and Mike just sat there staring at the menu. Every time the waitress came by, Ben would beg for her phone number. The flirtation was quite comical and completely innocent but I could see the wheels spinning in Kristi's head. I could also see her checking out the bus boy. Well, she was the one who just wanted to be friends, right?

I couldn't blame Ben for flirting with every woman that brushed by the table. That comment must have bruised his ego and Kristi wasn't exactly being Miss Personality. For the first time in a long time, I wasn't spending my evening lying on the bathroom floor and I was really enjoying talking to Ben. I, however, was not at all attracted to him. I was in such a state of gratitude, and thankful for everything, including meeting new people, having great conversation and…onion breath. Even though I wanted to keep my eye on the prize, the prize was contemplating whether to order extra cheese on his nachos.

As the evening wore on, I realized I had not been given a minute alone to talk to Mike. Something had to be done.

I moved in closer. Ben immediately slid in. I changed seats and Ben changed as well. At one point, he got up to go to the washroom, and I placed his drink and jacket beside Kristi. He came back and moved it. I could not get away from him. We were playing an adult version of duck, duck and goose.

By the end of the night, I had not reached my goal. Everybody went home and I went to the toilet.

The day before my next treatment, I was horny and frustrated. I knew it would be another three weeks before I could try again. I also felt very scared. Those few days of feeling good came and went so fast. Now I was entering the world of being a sickly cancer patient again.

The day before my chemo treatment was always the worst. It was important for me to eliminate any stress from my life and just relax and be calm and not take on other people's problems. Then the phone rang. It was Kristi.

"I have been giving this a lot of thought," she analyzed. "I haven't slept in days."

I knew exactly where this was going with this. She wanted to know where I bought my leather jacket.

"It's taken me a long time to bring this up because I know you have chemo tomorrow," she expressed.

She went on to accuse me of trying to steal her man. She couldn't trust me.

"How could you do this to me? I had friends like you in high school and I'm not doing it again." She continued, "All you care about is boys and I am way beyond that in my life."

I hung up the phone. Now let me explain. I felt like there was no point crying over the fact that I had cancer, and no amount of tears was going to make it better, or take it away. I had to deal with it and keep living my life. It was a speed bump. This conversation was one of the only moments I actually cried.

The next day I was lying in the hospital bed having treatment and my cell phone rang again. Kristi called again because she thought it would be a great time to allow me to "say my peace". I know she was looking for an apology.

"Do you have anything to say for yourself Ally?" she asked.

"Yes," I answered. "Did Mike ask about me?"

I realized that people's true colours are exposed when someone needs them the most. I also realized that I didn't need to keep the Preparation H for my eyes and my butt beside each other. I needed loyalty from the people in my life.

CHAPTER 10
The Healer and my Heart

Why did I get it? Why are others given skinny legs and a natural ability to whistle and, I got cancer? The facts are that I had no family history; I wasn't overweight (in medical terms. In my eyes, I was a work in progress) and I had a very healthy lifestyle (uh, wine is good for you). Was it being on the birth control pill for too long? If so, why didn't my doctors say something? Why did they keep handing out yearly prescriptions like it was hotel soap from Super 8? Was it the years of partying too much? If I knew I was going to get cancer, I would have partied more. Was it the diet foods? I'm sure carb free, sugar free, diet, low fat, no fat, flax seed and kefir enriched triple soy processed apple sauce six times a day was riddled with nutrients. Or was it trying to succeed, run a business, pay a mortgage, be thin, be fit, be wrinkle free, be happy, and be partnered off before Bridget Jones is a grandmother? Was it the stress of it all?

After one of my treatments, my friend Katia gave me a gift certificate to a new age healer. We met while working together at the acting school. Katia is from Slovakia and immigrated to Canada on her own, eventually becoming a citizen. Her determination inspired me. Both of our families lived far away, so we bonded and became each other's family. She is like a sister to me, borrowing my clothes and oversharing. We couldn't be more different. She believes in past lives and I believe in passing joints. She reads tarot cards, and I use them to pick my teeth. She has a very Zen approach to life and believes in alternative medical practice.

This particular healer practiced German New Medicine. The type of therapy she practices is called Body Talk. It is the belief that the body and mind are connected and your body is trying to tell you things that are going on in your mind. Body Talk taps into your body to heal the mind and vice versa. When I first met Val, the healer, I was very ill. She had a room inside a chiropractor's office and as I was sitting in the waiting room, I kept running to the bathroom to throw up.

Val was a very kind Polish woman with a thick accent and an even thicker moustache. She had me lie down on the table, put a barf bucket by my side, squeezed my forearm and began to talk. The combination of her simple touch and soft voice really calmed me down. I never barfed for the rest of the day.

She quietly asked me, "Vat kind of Ken Sar do vu heave?"

"Breast" I answered.

I felt like such a cliché. Of course I had breast cancer. I had boobs. Breast cancer was everywhere. I couldn't go into a store without seeing something that had a pink ribbon on it. From frozen dinners to rollerblades, everything was branded with that damn ribbon! What about the other cancers? What about my friend Steve, a business owner and champion skier who had just been diagnosed with jaw cancer? He had to get reconstructive surgery and it took him over two years to learn to talk again. What about eight year old Madison that had lymphoma and her parents had to quit their jobs so she could move into the city to get the proper treatment? What about her? What about my friend Janet's father that had cancer of the liver and died suddenly one year earlier? Where are all the frozen dinners and races for all of those heroes? I am not minimizing the disease or downplaying what I or any other breast cancer survivor has gone through. There is no doubt about it, it sucks, but it just seems that breast cancer was becoming a brand. Want to sell a computer? Slap a pink ribbon on it and you're the next Bill Gates! I asked myself why so many people were getting on the boob wagon and my male friend put it into perspective,

"Because everyone loves boobs; male or female, everyone wants to save them." Well, there it was! There's not a testicular cancer frozen dinner! Boobs are beautiful, balls are ugly.

I always got pissed off when I told someone I had breast cancer and their eyes would head straight to my tits.

"They're not going to fall off right in front of you," I thought.

I realized how much hell I went through to save them, so why should I be mad that they want to look?! I should be proud of my fun bags! So go ahead world and stare at my girls, stick your head right in my cleavage and motorboat them if you want to! Let my tits be your oyster!

Val then shook her head and said "Vat Brest in vit in?"

"The right," I answered.

"So vu had ver hart broken?"

"Yes," I said trying to stop the tears.

"Vit out any exvination? No veason. He just veft you?"

"Yes!" This time I couldn't stop the tears and just let them fall.

She squeezed my arm tighter, comforting me "And vis happened one vear or a vear and a half ago?"

"Yes," Oh god! How did she know this? Katia and I had just met recently through work and I didn't tell her about The Ass-Man. Quite frankly, I was just getting to a point in my life where I had finally let it go. There was no way she could have known this.

Val went on to explain to me that wherever your pain is located, is directly associated with something in your life. Since breast cancer is so close to the heart, she knew I had my heart broken. The right breast represents the loss of a relationship and the left breast represents the loss of a child. The loss of a child does not necessarily mean death, it could mean the child leaving the nest and going off to college, or getting married or distancing themselves from your life. Sure enough the more women I met, the more I realized that her theory could very well be true. She also knew it happened over a year prior because once the initial stress of it is over; the body takes a year or so to form the tumour. The stress is just the trigger to get things started. Not only did I have to live with the fact that I had my heart broken by a six foot man child, but that he also gave me cancer! I would have rather settled for his twenty unsold boxes of butt calendars. No, I'm wrong, there were twenty-eight boxes but I'm not petty.

I allowed this blame game to go on for quite a while. I needed to find a reason for my diagnosis and he was the target. After the pain subsided, I came to the realization that it wasn't him. He didn't tie me to a bed and inject a tumour into my boob. In fact, he never tied me at all. Total let down. Yes, he was a certifiable narcissist, spinning every situation on himself. During our relationship, I ran a very successful event for a local radio station. They were really impressed with my on air presence that I was immediately offered a job. Honoured, and of course flattered, I shared the news with him hoping he would agree with the sentiment.

"Did you ask about me?" he responded.

He always had to showcase how liked he was, presenting me with texts from other women wanting to meet him.

Although I wanted it to be, we were never on the same team.

I finally did get my closure with that relationship. He had called me after not speaking for over a year. I thought he was calling because he heard what had happened and wanted to wish me well. As it turned out, he did hear what happened. He had recently become a financial planner and needed to obtain some clients. He assumed I was dying and thought it would be a good time for me to invest. My crisis was his opportunity.

That action made me realize how grateful I was to have gone through it single. The thought of worrying about someone else's reaction to my treatment scares me more.

The fact of the matter was that I did have a great deal of support. The whole process solidified the importance of a strong network in my life. I believe that the best gift you can give is support and I do this with my friends and family in any way I can. That encouragement can make a person feel unstoppable.

If you take away anything from this book besides good wine suggestions, (Malbec) is to remember how good support feels and to always give it to others. The genuine words "I'm proud of you" and "I'm happy for you" can change someone's life. It changed mine. My parents have always been my biggest fans. As an adult, I think, "What would Mom and Dad think of me?" And it helps me form my actions; like deciding against funnelling a beer and trying slack-lining for the first time. Wine is better. I want them to be proud. I try to act with integrity. Sometimes I don't, especially after a long weekend camping trip with five empty bottles of wine in the back of my truck but I'm human. A human with red stained teeth and lips I may add. I could have chosen to blame the Ass-Man for the rest of my life but I chose not to. I chose to no longer be a drama queen. My life used to be full of drama; I chose to live my life with no blame on myself and on others.

Life is one giant lesson and it is up to you if you want to enrol. Oh, that's good! Someone put that on a t-shirt. If you make a million bucks, I won't blame you. I'll just take half.

CHAPTER 11
Top Ten Dating Tips from the Chem-Ho

I learned a lot about dating while living as my alter ego. My mojo morphed into nojo. I was like a pet dog that had been retrieving tennis balls for two hours straight; lying down on the ground, exhausted, full of slobber, with ten wet balls torn to shreds by my side. I was jaded, exhausted and uninterested. All I wanted to do was to hump an over-sized pillow and be in bed by 9pm. Here are the top ten things I learned about dating.

1. **Needy is greedy**. Men want to chase. Be busy. If you're readily available there is no chase. Nada. It is like running after a sloth on Valium. No excitement there. I once stared at a phone for two days straight. Needy. Don't do it. Nobody likes it and nobody

wants it. I don't even like it when my dog is needy. There is only so much of her rubbing up against my right calf I can handle. Whoever you are and whatever relationship you are in, nobody wants a needy partner. Unless it's George Clooney needing me in his Italian villa by noon tomorrow to rub his shoulders. That, I want. Don't cancel plans with your friends to meet a guy you just met swiping to the right because his profile picture is his face photo-shopped onto Dwayne Johnson's body. Don't wait by the phone. Don't look at your phone every five minutes. It is not going to turn into a giant penis with a big heart. Transformers haven't even figured that out yet and neither will you. Friendships are everything. Don't give that up for an idea. Believe me I know. I once stared at a phone so long that I was temporarily colour-blind.

2. **Stability is key**. If a guy isn't stable in his career, his finances, or his living situation, he won't be stable with you. He does not feel like a man yet. Men are essentially hunters and if they feel like they can't provide, they are not invested. And don't let him convince you that his basement apartment is only temporary. His parents live upstairs and he didn't

get his allowance after not cleaning his plate from last night's dinner. My theory is every family is crowned with a man-child and I've dated all of them. Don't go there. You can't change him. You can't tell him how to live. He needs to want it for himself. He won't do it for a girl he just met trolling the Internet. And, the only reason he contacted you on Facebook is because he wants to get down your pants. Don't see a man for his potential. See him for what he is right now. You can't change him.

3. **Find your passion and interests**. Know who you are and what excites you. Your passion is not dating. Your passion is not contacting exes on Facebook. I should know. I was blocked more times than I received new friend requests. I considered it a "special skill" that I could highlight on my resume. You have a better chance of meeting someone doing something you enjoy; whether it be artistic like joining a theatre group, or a sports league like toe wrestling. Couples that have common interests are more likely to last.

4. **A red flag is red for a reason**. In my case, those flags should have been on fire. If it feels like a red

flag then it is! It would be the only way to get my attention. If the person you are dating does not make you feel good, or makes you question yourself this is called A RED FLAG. Run far away and don't look back. Listen to your friends, they know. They want you to be happy. They also want you to quit borrowing their Jimmy Choo strappy sandals and buy your own.

5. **Look after yourself**. Avoid the bar scene. There is nothing attractive about someone vomiting jalapeno poppers into a beer jug with a lit cigarette poking out of their cleavage. I did that once and it did not end well. It all starts with you. Treat yourself how you would want to be treated. This includes negative self-talk, your diet and exercise and overall health.

6. **Let a man do things for you**. Since the beginning of time, men have been the hunters. They have also been leaving their dirty socks on the floor and not replacing the toilet paper. You can't change evolution. Being independent is great, but let them do what makes them feel like men. They already have a mom and she is already annoying, so don't become their backup. This was the biggest lesson for me.

I have been independent for so long that I pride myself in it. That and being able to put on a pair of Spanx with one hand.

7. **Get what you give**. If you want love, then you have to give it. You want a compliment, give one. Show appreciation. Smile. Be kind to people. Listen! I heard this quote the other day "The biggest problem we have is we don't listen to understand, we listen to reply". Yes that was me. If you truly want to get to know someone, then listen to them. Learn about them. Find out if he truly is a good match for you, instead of proving to him how good you are for him. You're not a used car salesmen, you're a person and you're pretty awesome!

8. **Avoid over-sharing.** Would you want to invest in a house if you learned the last owners used the kitchen floor as a toilet? There are things people just don't need to know. There is nothing appealing about bragging about ex-lovers, how drunk you got last weekend or that weird rash on your thigh. Avoid it.

9. **Know what you want**. How are you supposed to place an order if you don't know what you want? Write down your must haves and keep them with

you at all times. Write down five things that your ideal partner MUST HAVE. Next time you meet someone with potential, look at the list and if they don't meet all five, MOVE ON. I keep my list in my wallet on the back of a KFC receipt. It works. Here is an example of 5 MUST HAVES:

- Financially stable

- Physically fit

- Honest

- Likes to travel

- over 18

10. **Enjoy the ride.** Have fun! Dating should be fun, so enjoy it. If at first you don't succeed, remember you have learned something and you are one step closer meeting your ideal mate…or a restraining order.

CHAPTER 12
The Real Doctor and the chicken wings

My goals changed after getting diagnosed. Before cancer, I wanted to get married and have children. After cancer, I wanted to marry a doctor and have no hangovers.

I had been put under anaesthesia more times in one year than I had a banana shaped bowel movement; apparently the banana shape is the sign of a healthy digestive system. Mine resemble garden gnomes. The first time I was put under, the anesthesiologist came to chat with me right before surgery. My friend Janet and I were sitting in my hospital room laughing at a magazine they gave me that was for women over fifty when he walked in. I was a rarity in the breast cancer world. Most women who were diagnosed were over fifty and post-menopausal. I was part of the one percent of women in my age group that got breast cancer. I was also part of the one percent of women in my age group that wore blue mascara. Janet is also a rarity in the world. She is three years older than me but could pass off as fifteen years younger. That prediction was verified one night when we were invited to double date at a high school graduation. We had met two guys in a parking lot off of the busiest strip in town. They invited us into their minivan to smoke a joint (no inhaling) only for us to immediately discover that it belonged to their mother. They were staying out past curfew to cruise the strip for prom dates. I immediately obliged, as I took it as an opportunity to re-do my own horrific prom. My father drove me there dateless in his pyjama pants and walked me right to the punch bowl. My dress had the price tag intact hanging off the armpit as Mom hoped to return it the following morning. The only guy that asked me to dance was the janitor, or so I thought, but he wanted me to so he could mop. I needed a redo.

"He's as old as my son," Janet yelled yanking my head out of his chest.

"You could get arrested!" she warned as she pushed me out of the minivan.

I still managed to leave the scene with his phone number written on the back of a piece of sandpaper. I remember getting a rash on my chest after stuffing it in my bra.

Janet runs three successful businesses independent from her ultra athlete successful husband. She is a fabulous mother to three grounded and overachieving children and she still manages to look like she belongs on a red carpet. Janet is one of those women that people love to hate but you can't hate her, believe me, I've tried. She is a lot of fun, very creative and an amazing friend. When I got diagnosed, she rallied all of our friends together and every morning I would wake up with a new care basket on my doorstep. She was there for me as much as she could be, and with a family to run, she was there beyond any expectation.

This day, she was my wing woman when the handsome anesthesiologist entered the room. He was tall, with curly brown hair, dark skin, dark eyes, and a personality that lit up the room. According to the magazine I had been reading, my hot flashes could also heat up a room, so the two of us were on fire.

He asked me questions about my tolerance for drugs and I bragged about how I could drink him under the table. He snapped back with a witty comment about how he's woken up under a table a few times. I retorted with a comment about how I've woken up under a table in Vegas a few times. Now, I had been warned about anaesthesiologists. They are the one type of doctor you don't want to date. I beg to differ. I think the one doctor you don't want to date is Dr. Phil.

I liked the banter of the new doctor and I had it going on and I also liked that he kept talking to my chest. We talked about common interests, red wine and white wine. Then he said he had always wanted to be a comedian. I told him that I hosted an open mike comedy night every Sunday. He became very interested. Either that or he liked the fact that I wasn't wearing a bra.

He left the room and told me that he would definitely see me again in surgery. Janet and I gave each other a look and simultaneously reached for my chart to find more about my future husband. All we found was his signature, no name. The only letter we could make out was a D, for doctor. I called over the first nurse I saw, told her I had cancer and needed one last fling. She told me she was the coffee cart lady but hadn't been with a man since her divorce fifteen years prior, so she would be glad to help.

Tears started to well up in her eyes and we never saw her again. We never did get any coffee either.

I realized my only option was to make my move on the operating table. It wouldn't be the first time I had charmed a man while under the influence, lying on my back with my shirt open. I knew I had this covered.

Hours later, I woke up as I was being wheeled back from surgery. I looked up and the person who was wheeling me back was none other than the hot anaesthesiologist.

When he put me back into my room, Janet and the nurse were dumbfounded.

"Nice work," Janet said.

"How did you do that?" the nurse questioned. "They never bring you back to your room."

Although I don't remember what I said from the moment when he gave me the anaesthesia, I do remember the last thing he said when leaving:

"Tell your dad to stay away from your nightstand drawer. See you at comedy night."

Janet burst into laughter. Lying there in the operating room, I told my most personal and embarrassing story. Now I might as well tell you.

Ally Lane

First of all, I must start by saying that every time my parents come to visit, all they do is clean. They show up in radioactive outerwear: big rubber boots, gas masks, and Geiger counters. Mom carries a case of sticky notes and Dad is heavily masked and I can barely make out his voice as they bang on the front door.

"We are here," he breathed, sounding eerily like Darth Vader.

They immediately begin fumigating the house. My father's version of cleaning involves him spraying Lysol on everything.

"There is a smell coming from this corner." He walks towards the corner of my bedroom. "It's getting stronger." He moves closer, "I have located the smell," he says as he sprays an entire bottle in four squirts towards my dog.

"Congratulations Dad, you just located Peggy."

"Well she is sterile now," he rebuts while holding on to the waist of his pyjama pants as he feeds her a brick of cheese.

By the end of their visit my mother had decorated the entire house with post it notes, and has put half of my living room on the lawn labeled: FINAL SALE, MUST GO.

Once, I caught my dad cleaning off the neighbour's porch. My mother is all about the laundry. When I was a teenager she gave my friend and me a lecture on how to clean our jeans. "You have to smell the crotch, clean the crotch". I once found sticky notes on the crotch of every pair of my pants labeled: CLEAN.

My parents always go through everything I own. I throw out the garbage and my dad immediately dives in to go through it, as Mom figures out the resale value of every item.

When I moved, my dad came to help. Now we all know there are certain things, private things, things a single woman with a pulse needs to help her get through the day; things you don't want your father to find out about. While I was at work, my dad had eight hours alone to unpack, organize and clean. I had them carefully wrapped up in newspaper, covered in a black garbage bag and then duct taped three times over. I then hid them in a padlocked super steel box marked "Radioactive. Do not touch. You will die IMMEDIATELY." My dad called to say he had walked Peggy six times and he thought we should take her to the vet because she was sleeping too much. He then added that he only had one more box to unpack.

"Dear, do you have the key or should I use the pliers Mom packed?"

I screamed and hung up the phone, snuck out of work early through the bathroom window and ran down the street and knocked over a homeless man's house. I then missed the bus so I pulled a "Dukes of Hazard" through the passenger side of a recently imported cab belonging to a driver from Peru. "My dad is going to find my vibrator, this is an emergency. Step on it."

Thirty dollars later I blasted through the door, ran downstairs and saw the padlock on the floor; the box completely empty. I went through everything but couldn't find it, until three days later. All I can say is thank god my mother bought me a new shower-head.

Those were the worst three days of my life. I ripped the house apart; I couldn't sleep. I called into work sick. You could cut the tension with a Slap-Chop. Did he find it? Oh God! What if he did? What must he think of me now? I couldn't look him in the eye. All I could think about was that my dad now saw me as some kind of pervert. I wanted to die. On the day my father left, I decided to smooth the ice and make us a nice breakfast. When I was looking for a whisk I found it, my little friend freshly washed and put away... mistaken for an eggbeater. I don't know which is

worse, your battery-operated boyfriend being fou...
your father, or getting into a fight with the sales clerk ı
trying to return a used one.

The latter happened not too long ago. I had a few months of cancer therapy left before the end of my treatment process. My hair had grown into a funky short platinum blonde style and I was a spitting image of Pink. I just had my Port-o-Cath removed and I was able to wear any type of shirt I wanted again. I was working out every day while training for a cycling race that would wind through the Rocky Mountains. I was looking good and feeling great. Little did I know how great positive thinking and perseverance could be once I had met and fallen head over heels for a doctor; a real doctor, not someone who plays one on TV, although I wouldn't say no to Doogie Howser. That's right; the anesthesiologist who wheeled me back to my room post-op wasn't the first doctor I had ever fallen for.

His name was Matthew. He had seen my Chem-Ho videos and had sent me an email. "I think you're really pretty. Good luck finding a doctor". In order to be on YouTube, you must have a screen name and his was Cute Doctor. I couldn't believe my eyes. After creating over twelve videos searching for a cute doctor in the hospital, one came to me! I didn't even have to wait in the bushes outside his clinic.

He was a GP and worked as a consultant for a large multi-national company. He made up his own hours and only occasionally had to perform surgery. He was building a million dollar home on a few acres of land in The Rocky Mountains.

We had everything in common; we were born a day apart, we were from the same town, we were both ski instructors and had the same breed of dog.

We began talking over text message and he said he wanted to meet me after only our first conversation. Every day I would wake up with a message on my phone: "Can I meet you today?" He was very persistent. I was rather enjoying the chase so I kept him dangling for over a week, but by our first date, I couldn't wait any longer.

We met at a pub. From the moment I walked in and set my eyes on him, I knew he was the one. Let's face the facts, I am a chubby chaser and his stomach was hanging over his belt just the way I like it. He wore a baseball cap and I could tell by his profile that underneath it he must have had a shaved head. He looked absolutely adorable, just like the Pillsbury Dough Boy type I was attracted to. From the moment I sat down, the sparks were going like wild fire.

He was very funny and had a sarcastic wit about him that I liked. There was not a boring moment or a single lull in the conversation. He asked me questions that I know you are not supposed to ask on the first date but it felt so comfortable. He wanted to know about my past relationships and what I was looking for in one. I felt like I could tell him anything and so I did.

"Why are you still single?" he asked.

I always have dreaded this question because nobody had ever asked me and I wasn't sure how to answer. If someone had asked, I would have gladly obliged with an answer, but it had never come up before.

Before I could think of something funny to say, he answered for me. "I think it's because you're funny and you're hot. That intimidates men but I'm not intimidated."

He was very complimentary. He told me how he loved my style, loved the fact that I was always smiling, loved that I was so pretty. The compliments didn't stop. I was absolutely smitten.

By the end of the date he leaned in and said, "We should just get married." These were the words I had been waiting my whole life to hear and after 37 years, it had finally happened. It didn't feel awkward or creepy; it felt right. When I got home I immediately called my mother and told her I had just met the man I was going to marry.

There was silence on the other end. I didn't hear her voice for a long time until I realized she was crying.

"Why are you crying?"

"I am just so happy. I am so happy for you. You deserve this."

It was true. I did deserve this. I thought for a long time that I hadn't been given the chance at love because God had given me my life and I should be grateful for that. I had a wonderful family, great friends, an amazing career, and my health that I was so thankful for. Maybe love was demanding too much? Now that I was through with the worst part of my treatment and feeling terrific, God had given me what I wanted. It was all part of the divine plan and I was as happy as a dog that has just found a jar of peanut butter.

On our second date, we met at a pub. He told me he was crazy about me and asked if we could be exclusive. I said yes, and then I sat there as I watched him drink six beers, followed by three scotch chasers in under an hour.

I was mesmerized. He was absolutely amazing. He then got up and said he needed to get back to surgery. Later that night, I got a text message from him which read, "I love being with you." My heart melted.

For our third date, we met at a pub too. He told me that we should have our honeymoon in Whistler. He also felt it necessary to tell me that I had trust issues and I needed to see a psychiatrist. He assured me that seeing a shrink didn't make me a weak person. I thought about it and yes, maybe I did have trust issues. I know I got cancer from the stress of The Ass-man and it had taken me almost three years to get rid of him completely. I never sought counselling through all of this and the way I dealt with it was by making the YouTube videos. I thought about it further and maybe he was right. Finally, a man had come along and said something because he actually cared, not because he wanted something. He told me that date would have to be a quick one, as he had to go to work. He then ordered four scotches in a row and got into his car and drove. I missed him immediately as he drove away weaving in and out of the middle lane.

We saw each other as much as possible and as much as his busy schedule would allow. When we weren't together we were sexting. He missed me so much that he texted me right from the operating room and we talked about vibrators as a 70-year old woman was getting a hip replacement.

It bothered me that we had to always see each other around his schedule. I had to come to terms with the fact that I was dating a doctor and doctors are busy people.

He turned our courtship into a mysterious game; always meeting for short amounts of time, in dingy strip mall pubs. We would only talk over text message. He helped me with my trust issues assuring me that he wanted something real, reminding me not to close up my heart. He told me not to be jealous and insecure. He started saying that my behaviour was weird and I was scared to let him in. I thought I was just being cautious; after all, I had met him over the Internet. At this point I had not met any of his friends or seen where he lived and I was still trying to get to know him. I was in a constant struggle not to sabotage the one thing I had always wanted while also trying to keep my guard up. I frustrated him and as he took a swig of his scotch, he said, "Tell me what you want Ally. It's quite simple." I wanted it to work, I wanted to fall in love and get married. I didn't want to be alone anymore.

I decided to let my guard down and him get to know the real me. I marched right over to the sex shop, slapped my credit card on the counter and ordered up a pair of matching vibrators, a blow up doll, a mouth gag and swing. Since we had spent all of our time at my house, I thought I'd surprise him with a visit to his place with a treasure trunk full of surprises.

As soon as I mentioned I was coming over, everything went sideways. He attacked me over text message. I begged him to call me, as there must have been some misunderstanding. He ended our relationship right then and there over text. "It's official. It's over. Your crazy." I was completely shocked. How can a doctor not know how to spell you're correctly?

I called him immediately and his phone went straight to voicemail. I know I was born with a permanent foot in my mouth but this time I knew I hadn't said anything wrong. I went over and over the conversation in my head for about twenty times. How could a surprise visit to his house quantify an ending to our engagement and warrant my diagnosis as crazy?

A month, a mixed tape and a tribute video later, I realized he wasn't calling me back. I also realized that I had five hundred dollars' worth of his and hers sex toys.

I couldn't look at that vibrating devil in the face so I marched right back to the sex shop and demanded my money back. The clerk, a four-foot tall woman with a beard stared at me coldly.

"Hun, read the sign," she said strongly.

I followed her stubby fingers to the bright red sign hanging over the vibrating eggs. NO RETURNS, NO REFUNDS.

As I tried to explain how the toys had been unopened, I looked down at the counter and saw none other than my ex-boyfriend's naked butt staring right up at me. His ass modelling days had moved right into the butt plug market. I started to cry right there in the middle of the store during a blow up doll demonstration. I told her my whole sob story but she wouldn't budge. I was desperate. I had no choice but to pull out the cancer card. She pulled out the mace, and I was gone. I now had two new eggbeaters to add to my kitchen drawer.

Once I was tired of eating omelettes every morning, I ventured out to meet some friends for lunch. As I awaited my basket of fries, I heard a familiar voice shouting from the kitchen.

"Tell my wife I'll call her back. It's wing night for Christ's sake!"

I turned around where I had a clear view of the kitchen. Right there, frying up some wings was my doctor. I found out that I wasn't in love with a rich doctor but a bald and married fry cook at Hooters.

I realized I needed to rethink my dating goals. I also needed to rethink my choice in lunch places. After that, I had the runs for two days.

CHAPTER 13
The List

After my tryst with the Hooters cook, I decided I needed to make a change with my dating approach. At this point I was recovering from treatment, and I no longer wished to identify myself as the Chem-Ho. That was "her" wish; a way to enjoy the hospital visits instead of dread them. I had to shed "her" skin, begin the healing process.

The Chem- Ho was a crutch. Nobody has control over cancer. It is not something anyone can fix, like a relationship or a car that keeps breaking down. It was out of my control. The one thing I could be in control of was her. It was in her hands. I couldn't be Ally controlling the cancer; I had to be someone else. She was my way of keeping Ally safe and free of destruction. It was empowering to know I didn't have to live this shit as Ally. It was so freeing to know I could put it in someone else's hands. I protected myself. It wasn't a big deal because I was in complete control. I was the director of the show.

The most drastic action I took post cancer was deleting my YouTube account and in the process, the 13 volume series. It was now lost in cyberspace, never to be located again.

Now I didn't need her anymore. It was time to break up. I was ready to move on. I went through all the stages of loss; denial, anger, bargaining, depression and even a few more like wine, beer, scotch, and back to wine. I was now in the final stage, acceptance. I was ready to get on with my life as Ally, finding a doctor to date was not a priority whereas it was the Chem-Ho's ONLY priority. I didn't NEED a doctor anymore. I needed someone stable in all areas of my life.

After all the counselling and the constant reciting of lines to <u>The Secret</u>, I realized I was not going to get what I wanted, unless I asked for it SPECIFICALLY. My therapist suggested I make a list. I kept that list and hung it on the wall of my home office. I will share it with you now. Keep in mind she told me to be specific.

The Chem-*HO*

1. Male. (To quote my therapist: "What if you ask for all these specific traits and you receive them, but it's a donkey?")

2. 35-38 years old. (I was 37 when I wrote this. I figure the age is a good compromise, the wrinkles have not set in and sunblock is retroactive).

3. Latin. (What can I say? I love Latin men. Plus, I want to learn conversational Spanish).

4. Dark hair.

5. Dark eyes.

6. Physically fit.

7. Strong. (I can't lift everything myself. Well, I can, but I don't want to. I like to get my nails done).

8. Sexy. (A nice body but not all muscle and no fat. I don't want to cuddle a rock formation).

9. Good teeth. (Or good dental insurance.)

10. Soft skin. (Not soft from eating three pizzas kind of soft.)

11. Between 5"9 and 6"2. (Short man syndrome is a real thing people!)

12. A good lover. (Let me be the judge of that.)

13. A great communicator. (I want to know where I stand and where he stands, like on top of a wedding cake.)

14. Financially stable. (Has a steady job and not one that involves an allowance from his live in mother.)

15. A great sense of humour and loves to laugh. (With me, not at me, unless I am attempting to ride a horse.)

16. Honest. (Yes I do look fat in those pants.)

17. He has goals and dreams. (Real future goals and not ones like taking a hit off a bong without coughing.)

18. Active. (Must be a good surfer, mountain biker and snowboarder.)

19. Adventurous. (Not the kind that involves another couple and a swing.)

20. Emotionally stable.

21. Loves dogs and owns a Labrador retriever. (I'm a dog person but he has to be a big dog person. A man with a small lap dog is questionable.)

22. Drives a white Tacoma truck. (Hey, you've got to throw the dog somewhere and I've always wanted a white Tacoma.)

23. Supportive. (Of me, and my career.)

24. Creative. (But not in the same industry as me. One insecure person in the relationship is enough.)

25. Close with his family. (Well, if he is Latin, we've got that covered. His family cannot be living in the same house as him.)

26. He accepts and loves my family. (If he can buy my dad some new pyjama pants, that's a plus.)

27. Eats right. (You know that phrase 'You are what you eat'. I don't want a man that looks like a deep-fried perogy.)

28. Likes to travel. (And not out of state type traveling because of a warrant.)

29. Independent. (And encourages me to be, but not "get out of the house so I can hit on your friend" type encouragement.)

30. Integrity.

31. Wants to get married. (Not in a "someday when hell freezes over" kind of way. I chose the spot I want to get married: on the beach in Sayulita, Mexico. So the wedding planning is already done. I'm efficient.)

32. Faithful.

33. Happy with himself. (And happy with me.)

34. Fun.

35. Likes to cook.

36. Handy.

37. Kind.

38. Considerate.

39. Sociable.

40. Available.

The latter is ode to the Hooters cook. I learned my lesson there. It's important to be specific. When I presented this to my therapist she was shocked. She was expecting a list of maximum ten things but mine was a tall order. (See number 11)

I've been through a lot in my life and I have learned and I have grown. Making this list was important to me. I believed in it and I believed in myself. I had earned this man. I knew he was out there. Wherever he is, he is certainly not deep-frying jalapeño poppers on game night. So come and get me, I am ready. Seriously I'm ready. Hurry; I have to pee and I feel a sneeze coming on.

CHAPTER 14
HOT FLASH

After a cornucopia of bad boyfriends, choices, and premature trauma (and a few other incidents of prematurity), I sit here at the bar with my two broken hands, and have come full circle. I've developed the tools to deal with whatever life throws at me including the value of laughing at it all. Let's face it; two broken hands are nothing but funny until I have to go to the washroom in a pair of Spanx.

I've realized my overall health and wellbeing is more important to me than anything else. "Who cares that I can't fit into a size two? I'm alive!" I proclaim chugging a Baileys on ice as the cube lodges in the back of my throat. I spent most of my life hating my body. Now I need to celebrate all that it has done for me. Why should I complain about a fat arse when those cells kept me alive when I couldn't eat for a week? Why should I complain about my thick legs when they trekked through hundreds of miles in a cycling race a week after my last chemotherapy? And most of all, I will never be ashamed of who I am and where I came from because those experiences made me who I am. I am proud of who I am. I beat cancer for f*8k sake! I'm awesome! It is time to celebrate my body and my spirit instead of fighting against it. During treatment, I began a new chapter in my life. I studied and became a certified fitness trainer and nutritionist. I began working, teaching at boot camps and as a trainer at a women's gym. This was a huge step for me as I was never an athlete growing up and I never viewed myself as the Jillian Michaels type. The clients did not want that anyway. They wanted someone real who could make them feel good. In the process they made me feel good too. I have made some lifelong friends in the process of my health recovery including the beautiful gal that is editing this book. Hey Lauren, try not to "accidentally" drive over this chapter again. Through everything, I found my purpose; nothing brings me more happiness than helping others discover their joy. It is so infectious.

As a sit here in two casts, pondering my life, I realize I have a giant grin on my face. I don't know if it's me, the wine buzz or the fact that the cute Latin guy has come back to talk to me.

"Sorry I left you sitting all alone. Those were old friends from high school I haven't seen in a while."

He proceeds to tell me he recently moved back from London, England after six years abroad. He missed his friends and family. It feels so good to finally talk to a man I'm not trying to impress. I can be so real with him. We talk about traveling, our goals in life and we laugh. "I'm so tired of dating losers, all I want is to sit on a beach, surf and write". All of a sudden his demeanour changes and his face changes to a pale white.

"Sorry, do you have a thing for losers?" I groan.

"You have no idea what you have just said to me right now," he steps back.

Oh, crap NOW! What have I said? Maybe he just broke up with his boyfriend who was born on a beach?

"Do you have kids?" he asks.

I think to myself, "Good retort," as this is such a loaded question. Now, 'HE has no idea what he has just said to me right now.'

I pray he doesn't continue with the follow-up, "Do you WANT kids?"

That is the question that constitutes a very long winded answer followed by a scotch chaser, a few tears and probably the end of this very enjoyable repartee. I have to find a way to steer this conversation back on track. I also have to find a way to stop the urge to pee as my Kegels are working on overdrive.

The chemotherapy was extremely rough on my body with varying side effects I did not predict. At the height of my treatment, I was on 14 different types of medication to strictly manage those; mouth sores, haemorrhoids and Neupogen. Ah yes, I haven't even written about the Neupogen yet, have I?

Chemotherapy can mess with your white blood cell count. Those cells fight off infections in your body like a common cold. If your cell count is low, you are at a very high risk of developing an infection that can become fatal. Before treatment began, I underwent a series of tests to monitor my white cell count. It was during this time the doctors uncovered an illness I had been living with undetected my entire life. My white cell count (neutrophil levels) was shockingly low for no explained reason. After several visits with a haematologist and a self-diagnosis of leukaemia, thanks Web MD, I was properly diagnosed with Cyclical Neutropenia. I was the first patient they had ever met with this disorder. "You are as special as a snowflake," the Haematologist muttered as I tried to rub her intern student's thigh under the table. The only way to boost the white cell count in order to qualify for chemotherapy was a drug called Neupogen. I was ordered to inject a dose of the drug into my stomach whenever my count was low. This meant daily visits to the cancer ward to administer blood tests to check the count. Then back home to await the call of the results. If the count was too low, I was asked to inject myself. Then back to the hospital to check the count again and so on and so on. I felt like I was on a Merry-Go-Round in a Walmart parking lot in the shittiest town in the world. To top it all off, the drug was not covered under any health care plan. Each vial cost approximately $400 and depending upon my level, injections could be up to five times a week. Drugs are so expensive. No wonder in high school we used to simulate the experience of getting high by staring into the flood lights of the Parliament Buildings. After staring into the lights straight on for five minutes, everything appeared purple. It was called a "Visit to Purple City". For some reason, I don't think a flood light high would work in my case. If the doctors could not control my white cell count, I could not receive chemotherapy and if I could not receive the therapy I could not meet any hot doctors. It was an Elizabethan tragedy. One day, the nurse on my team applied for my acceptance into a clinical trial. Much to my surprise, I was accepted and the drug was free. Why can't they have clinical trials for wine clubs?

I was off to the races and off to meet my future husband but after a few months, the blood disorder became the least of my worries. I began to experience waves of intense heat that would come out of nowhere like a flash followed by a wave of intense cold. It almost felt like a panic attack or a reverse orgasm. I don't even know what the latter is.

I decided to pay a visit to my oncologist. When I arrived, she asked me if I was still having my period. This was something I completely forgot about due to my abundance of health mishaps.

She looked at my chart and then spoke quickly like a hiccup, "Oh you're in menopause." I think she could tell by the look on my face that I was not informed this would transpire. What followed was the most inappropriate tagline a single woman wants to hear, "You froze your eggs, didn't you?" My heart sank into my half-boobed right chest, "No. No, I didn't."

"I'm sure I told you to freeze them," she replied.

She told me a lot of things but I don't recall most of them. I was in a haze of disbelief, of shock, of bewilderment and of denial. I was a self-employed, single woman living alone with cancer. I had so much to deal with that even if she did tell me, having children was so far down my list of priorities that it did not even register. She warned me of a whole list of things. She told me I had cancer. She told me I would lose my hair. She told me to buy a wig. She told me I would get very sick. I would need care. I couldn't do it on my own. I needed treatment; 27 rounds of two different chemo concoctions, and 20 rounds of radiation. I needed an operation. She used terminology I didn't understand; I wouldn't understand. I had no family history and no exposure to this world. I was just a number to her. I was like a cow awaiting slaughter; in and out of her office as fast as I could go. My head was overloaded with information and I was just trying to stay afloat. I had a business to run, bills to pay and an overly dramatic family to look after. I had to stay sane for them, for my friends, for myself. So EXCUSE ME if egg freezing was not at the top of my priority list. That was HER job, not mine! Almost all of her patients were post-menopausal and had no interest in conceiving. She could have simply missed informing me of this utterly important piece of information.

"Ugh, maybe I missed telling you that but everybody knows your chances of having a fertile egg after chemo is next to impossible."

Everybody does not know that! I didn't. Nobody told me, Now what do I do?

"Ally, you could sue," my counsellor suggested.

For what? To get my eggs back?

What sort of stress would that manifest in an already stressful world that I'm trying to manage? At 37, I was already considered a high risk for having a child, and now I have completely eliminated my chances of ever having a child of my own.

"What about adopting a Chinese baby?" my counsellor barked.

The truth was I didn't want a baby on my own. I wanted to be loved. I wanted a man to hold me in his arms and tell me everything was going to be OK. He would love me no matter what. Now, who is going to love me now? Who wants an infertile 37-year-old woman with no hair, half a boob, carrying around a barf pail, having hot flashes, haemorrhoids and growing a moustache like a bitter grandmother sitting on a front porch yelling at the mailman. What sort of lesson is this? What on earth did I do to deserve this? I don't deserve this cruelty. I did not sign up for this. I don't want this life. This life is pointless. I'm useless!

So when I'm asked about children, excuse me if it takes me a second to answer but before I can, he answers for me.

"I don't have kids either. I don't think I want them. I'd rather have a beautiful woman by my side I can travel with."

"But I thought you were gay," I said dumbfounded.

He rolled his gorgeous brown eyes, "No, I'm Andre; nice to meet you."

CHAPTER 15
Conquered it all!

As I lay here on the beach in Cabo Mexico writing the final chapter of this book, I take in deep breath of gratitude; I am grateful for my health. I am now nine years cancer free. I am grateful to everyone at The Tom Baker Cancer Centre for taking such good care of me, for laughing at my jokes, for wiping my butt, and enduring almost two years of a video camera being shoved in their face without complaint. Ok, I may have heard a few complaints, but they really should lock the men's urinals. I fought hard to save my breasts, and because of that, I wear them like medals. I'm no longer ashamed of my body, especially my boobs. If an admirer wants to examine them further, I won't stop them. My boobs are the world's boobs! Feel them up, feel them down and feel them all around. Do the hokey-pokey and turn my nipples around. That's what it's all about. Could you imagine if I had cancer of the clitoris? Actually nobody would be able to find it.

I'm proud to say I'm the healthiest I have ever been, inside and out. Even though I know in my heart there is nothing wrong, I still worry when I attend my yearly check-ups. I think that is a fear that will never go away. Last week my heart took a nosedive when I found a black lump on my neck. Deja Vu kicked in as I made the rounds of doctor appointments. The diagnosis came immediately; the lump was a ball of black mascara from neglecting to wash my face for weeks on end. The fear of reoccurrence will never quite go away because cancer does not discriminate. It can happen to anyone. The one thing I've learned is that I can only control my thoughts and reactions. I'm getting a lot better at it but I'm still a work in progress. When you face your own mortality, the little things don't seem to matter anymore. When the waitress delivers me the wrong order, I don't take it personally. I just don't tip. Now that's progress.

I've learned you have to be an advocate for your own health. You have to be your biggest support system and cheerleader. Nobody can take better care of you than yourself, including your mental health. I don't beat myself up anymore, unless I'm attending Ninja Warrior fitness classes. I try not to be too hard on myself. Laughter saved my life and I try to laugh as much as possible, looking for the funny in everything. My guilty pleasure is watching re-runs of Law and Order SVU. Realizing that is not a funny show, there is plenty to laugh at, especially Ice T's acting. There is so much pain in the world, especially right now, that I refuse to suck myself into the negative. I choose laughter. I choose fun.

As the Chem-Ho, my objective was to find love. What I realized was that my objective was already in front of me the whole time. I had a lot of love in my life. I never realized how much I was loved by those around me. I never realized how impactful I could be on my community and on others. I was honoured to be an advocate for cancer awareness and living life with positivity and laughter. My relationship with my family has never been stronger. It really brought us together and I love them for all their flaws and hang ups. I learned to embrace my mother's frugality and my dad's fashion sense. He gave up on the pyjama pants. Spandex is much more practical. My siblings and I have bonded. This summer, we organized our parents' 50th wedding anniversary party. It was a beautiful celebration that we will always remember fondly. Especially Mom, she has frozen all the leftovers.

My friendships are very important to me. I've learned that life is way too short for toxic relationship. A person's character is exposed not only when something tragic happens but more so when something good happens. I'm proud of my friends and they are proud of me. There is enough in this world for everyone. We all need to remember that.

I look out onto the ocean waves to admire my husband, Andre, surfing another wave. Allow me to rephrase that, shredding a wave. He is a fantastic surfer. Who would have thought I'd meet a Latin surfer in landlocked Alberta, Canada? We are a fifteen hour drive from the Pacific Ocean. Actually, I thought of it! I asked for it. I manifested it. He is everything on my list except for #11, height. For that, I am willing to compromise. We are the same height which has its advantages. I don't have to move the seat back when I get into his truck. And yes, it is a white Tacoma. We purchased it after we got married in Sayulita, Mexico. The place I dreamed of tying the knot to unanimous response from friends, "AS IF".

Andre is my perfect fit. I express my gratitude for him every single day. But, you know what? I earned it. I waited a long time to meet him and went through a lot. Everything I endured brought me to him. I was meant to meet him at that moment. If I did not experience the childhood I did, I would never have moved two provinces away to start afresh. If I did not experience breast cancer, I would never have decided to date younger men. If I never would have decided to charge my mountain bike off the cliff to impress a boy, I would never have ended up in the pub that night feeling sorry for myself wearing two casts. And if it weren't for those broken hands, Andre never would have approached me and asked for the story. I'm not mad at the Australian boy for forcing me to ride that stunt. I'm so grateful to him. It all led me to my dream man and my dream life. And, just so we're on the same page, he is not gay. He was so compassionate that I thought for sure he must be. Boy, was I wrong? He can leave the house with stains on his shirt and not even flinch.

When Andre and I first started dating, I couldn't even feed myself. I'll leave my bathroom visits up to your imagination. Pause. Good visual? Sorry about that. Yes, I'm Canadian, obligated to insert an "I'm sorry" before the end. Andre insisted on helping me for the first few weeks cutting my food, driving and all the things that involve hands- basically everything. I couldn't. At first, it was embarrassing but I soon began to appreciate the gestures. When my hands finally healed up, I kept allowing him to help me. It felt good. I didn't need to be totally independent all the time. I realized that men want to feel needed. If they truly care about you, this is how they express their love.

We cannot have children of our own and decided not to adopt. We have decided child free is the path for us. We want to be the best aunt and uncle we can. Everyone has a different path in life and we must respect each other's choices. We must stop comparing ourselves to others. There are 7 billion people on this earth with 7 billion different lives. No one is better than the other. That is what makes us unique. Andre and I have decided to travel, explore other cultures, and learn from each other.

I found my perfect love and I believe everyone deserves romantic love. I refuse to believe that some people don't find it. You can. There is someone out there for everyone. I look at some people and I think, "How were they able to find someone?" But they did. Everybody has that certain someone. It doesn't matter if you have missing teeth or cellulite or listen to Nickleback, there is someone for everyone. Everyone deserves love. That is guaranteed. Open your heart and it will come.

This book was complete in 2010 but something in my heart told me not to release it to the world. I didn't feel it had a happy ending. I picked it up a year ago, and started again. I have grown so much since then, back when I was in the throes of recovery. I believe everything in life is an opportunity to grow and to learn. I still had a lot of learning to do. Today, I'm in the throes of life of enjoyment. I have my happy ending. It's not over yet and I'm excited to experience what is next for me. Right now, I'm excited to catch this wave with the love of my life. I got to go. Surfs up! Let's laugh together again soon.

CPSIA information can be obtained
at www.ICGtesting.com
Printed in the USA
LVOW03s0430020218
565001LV00001B/1/P